Administrative Leadership in Health, Kinesiology, and Leisure Studies

Developed by the
College and University
Administrators Council of the
American Association for
Active Lifestyles and Fitness

Editors
James E. Bryant
San Jose State University, Retired
Barbara A. Passmore
Indiana State University

KENDALL/HUNT PUBLISHING COMPANY
4050 Westmark Drive   Dubuque, Iowa 52004

President and Chief Executive Officer   Mark C. Falb
Vice President and Executive Director   Emmett Dingley
Continuing Education Editor   Bridget Hollick
Vice President, Production Editorial   Ruth A. Burlage
Production Editor   Charmayne McMurray
Cover Design   Deb Howes
Manufacturing Coordinator   Thomas Mai

Cover photo: Rodin, Auguste
              The Burghers of Calais (F1929-7-129)
              Rodin Museum, Philadelphia: Gift of Jules E, Mastbaum

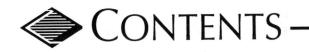 CONTENTS

Section I Understanding the Academy

Section II Realities and Theories of Managing and Leading

ABOUT THE COVER IMAGE

The cover sculpture, *Burghers of Calais*, was created by Auguste Rodin (1840-1917) in 1884 as a result of a request by the city of Calais. Calais wanted a monument to its heroic forefathers. As the story goes, there was an invasion of Calais, France and the city was surrounded. The invaders threatened to destroy the city. The Burghers, the city's administrators, offered their lives in return for the safety of the city. They were put to death and the city was spared.

Even though as an artist, Rodin is viewed as one who broke away from the high-minded academic standards that dominated French art since the 17th century, his work was selected by the editors of this book as representing the quandary in which administrators often find themselves. While department chairs are often referred to as neither faculty nor pure administrators, they are often compelled to break from tradition to represent faculty views to higher administration often putting themselves at great risk.

Deans, too, are often daring figures in the arena of fund development, faculty development and innovative administrative practices. Like Rodin, they often seek to reject the prevailing dogma of academic thinking in order to establish new paradigms of collegiality. Whether administrators using this text ever accomplish the equivalent of Rodin's great independent work—*The Thinker*—or whether they simply provide good solid leadership as a result, both have the potential to make a difference in people's lives.

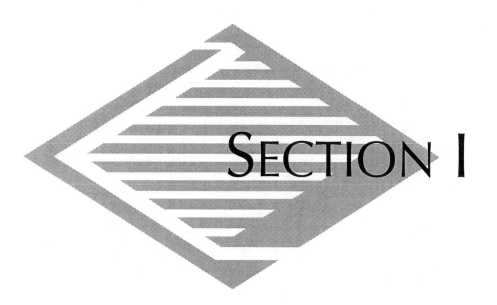

SECTION 1

Understanding the Academy

1 Promoting Health, Physical Education, and Recreation among Key Decision-Makers

John M. Dunn, *Dean and Professor, College of Health, University of Utah*

In accepting an administrative appointment, remember your roots, the things that initially "drove" you into higher education: a passion for teaching, a sense of wonderment and the scholarly, inquiring mind.

John M. Dunn

One of the challenges facing administrators in health, physical education, and recreation (HPER) units is how to communicate the role of these units within the overall mission of the institution to key decision-makers such as government officials, presidents, provosts, and trustees. The perception of HPER units and their value to higher education has varied through the years (Singer, 1998). In the 1960s, higher education was in a growth mode, with new buildings, expanding enrollments, and budgets that included incremental and predictable increases. Most disciplines planned with an eye toward expansion, and there were few, if any, conversations about program reductions or eliminations.

In the 1970s, the United States experienced an economic recession with severe budgetary implications for both public and private institutions of higher education. Budget shortfalls led policy-makers both within the academy (faculty senates, presidents, provosts) and external to it (trustees and legislators) to discuss the viability and importance of various departments and programs, with outcomes such as departmental and college mergers and reductions, and, in some instances, elimination of units in HPER (Ellis, 1998).

Ever since this painful period, many in higher education have had to reassess their priorities and ask challenging questions about the mission of various departments, including units in HPER. Recently, Jack Wilmore chaired a committee for the American Academy of Kinesiology and Physical Education (AAKPE) that asked members of the Academy to identify those characteristics of a HPER department that are most crucial to its survival (Wilmore, 1998). As noted in his article and supported by others whose views were reported in the same 1998 issue of *Quest*, many valuable lessons have been learned. The intent of this chapter is to identify some of the practical strategies that can be used to help decision-makers accurately—and, hopefully, favorably—assess the importance of HPER to institutions and to the people who are served by its programs.

Today, there is much good news about our field—about what we offer and how responsive we have been in expanding our mission to respond to various societal needs. The mission of most HPER units has broadened from its primary focus on preparing health and physical education teachers and community recreation personnel to identifying, nurturing, and creating new professional roles and career opportunities (e.g., fitness leaders; clinical exercise specialists; personnel focused on the needs of the elderly and individuals with disabilities). The nature and quality of our research has changed, with colleagues competing successfully for grants from prestigious federal agencies such as the National Institute of Health and the National Science Foundation to selected private foundations such as the Multiple Sclerosis Society and the American Dietetics Association. In addition, many of our units have recognized what Lawson (1999) refers to as our "social responsibility" and are responding to the needs of our communities, targeting specific populations that are underserved with intervention strategies designed to increase physical activity, reduce substance abuse, and provide nurturing environments for youths, the homeless, and the elderly. We also have benefited from and contributed to the increasing public interest in health, physical activity, and leisure (Dunn, 1998, 1999).

According to Morgan (1998), much of the renewed interest in what we do and offer has been kindled by several factors, including: publication of the encyclopedic volume, *Physical Activity, Fitness, and Health* (Bouchard, Shephard, & Stephens, 1994); the emphasis placed on physical activity in the release of *Healthy People 2000* (U.S. Department of Health and Human Services, 1990); the influence of the Centers for Disease Control and Prevention and their interest in and support for physical activity; and the publication of *Physical Activity and Health: A Report of the Surgeon General* (U.S. Department of Health and Human Services, 1996). The Surgeon General's report (SGR), a product of years of research relating physical inactivity to increased mortality and morbidity and reduced quality of life (Morrow and Blair, 1999), highlighted the significance of physical activity in overall health status. The SGR identified specific goals for the years 2000 and 2010 that governmental officials, professionals in higher education, and others should use to enhance the overall health of the general population.

Of course the information reported in the SGR is not new to professionals in HPER, who have argued for many years that the work they do is essential to the larger needs of society. Given the impetus of the SGR and other positive indicators supporting the value of physical activity and health, and the increasing proportion of seniors in our society, leaders of HPER units should be in an opportune position to advance their programs within their institutions (Wilmore, 1998). Morgan (1998) argued that "it is difficult to imagine a time in the history of our field, with the possible exception of the physical fitness movements resulting from the 'big' wars, when there was more public awareness and sensitivity regarding the importance of habitual physical activity" (p. 142). Given reports of an impending health crisis and the dramatic shift in the demographics of our population, the opportunities for promoting HPER units are exciting and positive.

Regardless of whether times are good or bad, or adequate funding is available or not, it is essential that department chairs and deans be vigilant in their efforts to promote their units so that decision-makers will value these units and their importance to their institution. At its annual gathering in 1998, AAKPE devoted its meeting to the theme of "Telling Our Story." The program was outstanding, with many helpful suggestions provided by thoughtful, knowledgeable, and experienced individuals. There were also cautionary words offered by a university chancellor (Portch, 1999) that "our story" is difficult to define because we have not identified a single, unified story for HPER. Others argued, however, that we have many stories to tell and that this is a desirable situation, given the range in size and mission of institutions that house HPER units (Franks, 1999). This latter philosophy will be incorporated into the suggestions that follow. Conveying what is important about your HPER unit must be positioned in the context of priorities that drive your state and region as well as the mission and strategic plan for your institution. The suggestions that follow will identify many of the strategies that have been used successfully by HPER program administrators to build and sustain outstanding programs. Not all of the suggestions will work in all settings, but they do represent positive ideas that will help to convey the importance of your HPER unit to key decision-makers.

Chairs and deans of HPER units must be interested in and must comprehend issues facing higher education in general (Kranebuhl, 1998). Establishing a knowledge base of topics in higher education will allow HPER administrators to anticipate and be conversant within discussions led by presidents, provosts, deans, and faculty leaders. This knowledge base will also allow administrators to convey their interest in broad issues confronting higher education and their willingness to add suggestions that might help their institution address these issues. Some current issues that are on the radar screen of most presidents and provosts include access, increasing diversity, containing costs, minimizing tuition increases, enhancing undergraduate education, using technology, distance education, accountability, faculty roles and rewards, university-community partnerships, and engagement.

Understand Broad Issues Confronting Higher Education

Information about these issues can be obtained from several sources. Depauw (1998) suggested that HPER administrators attend regional and national conferences sponsored by the American Association of Higher Education (AAHE), the American Council on Education (ACE), and the American Association of Colleges and Universities (AAC&U). Christina (2000) suggested that it is in the meetings and proceedings of AAHE where new trends that will affect HPER are identified and discussed, with solutions proposed by presidents, provosts, and deans. He adds that for HPER administrators not to be closely connected with AAHE is a serious mistake. Another excellent means of quickly obtaining information about current issues in higher education is to read the *Chronicle of Higher Education*. The electronic version of the *Chronicle* can be accessed daily, with an eye toward those topics that appear to be the issues of greatest concern to a particular institution. Campus leaders are impressed by chairs and deans who are interested in and conversant with topics that affect the larger institution. Knowing about such topics will go a long way toward establishing your credibility as an engaged administrator who can think beyond his or her own specific needs. Offering advice and suggesting solutions also helps to show others that HPER administrators are intelligent and creative.

Know Your Local Campus

Closely related to broad issues affecting higher education is the need to understand the local campus and its politics, leaders, priorities, and strategic initiatives. This can be accomplished in several ways, from studying the institution's mission statement to faithfully participating in campus-wide meetings (e.g., faculty or academic senate proceedings). In addition, the HPER administrator must become very familiar with the institution's policies and procedures, including its various curricula and faculty codes. For example, in response to program reductions in the 1970s and '80s, many institutions now have a policy related to program reduction or elimination. This policy—which many have found to be extremely important during budget crises—carries different names (e.g., San Jose State University uses the title "Academic Priorities Planning Process") (San Jose State University, 2000). While the policy varies from institution to institution, the criteria employed in making decisions about program reductions, eliminations, or enhancements normally focus on program centrality and quality, student demand, and future directions. As will be discussed later, it is essential that the mission statement of a HPER unit demonstrate a connection to the mission statement of the institution. Mission alignment can be accomplished by helping to create or shape the institution's mission or by developing a HPER statement that conforms to the institution's existing statement.

Furthermore, accepting roles and responsibilities on strategic committees helps to ensure that your unit's voice is heard and allows others to acknowledge and appreciate your initiative and leadership. These settings can also help you build personal relationships that may be critical in the future. There is no substitute for personal contact—for getting to know someone and finding common ground—when you are facing a major confrontation related to budget decisions, curricular infringement, or other equally challenging or sensitive issues.

Develop a Strategic Plan

Successful academic units employ a strategic plan that communicates—both internally and externally—their future directions and priorities. Such a document is very important in helping to establish a connection to the institution's overall priorities and objectives. An appropriate plan demonstrates how educational programs, research, and outreach activities offered by the HPER unit contribute to the institution's mission (Scanlan, 1998).

Although various techniques can be used to develop a plan, an analysis of the unit's strengths, weaknesses, opportunities, and threats (commonly referred to as a SWOT analysis) will provide a solid foundation for the unit's mission statement and specific objectives for a defined period of time (normally three to five years). SWOT analysis should include input from all stakeholders within the unit to ensure that the strategic plan is understood and widely adopted. It is also important to identify a faculty member or administrator—preferably someone external to the unit—to serve as a facilitator during this analysis. This individual will have a unique opportunity to become familiar with the HPER unit, its administrators, and faculty, and may later become one of the unit's strongest supporters.

Once the strategic plan is developed, the document should be shared widely within the institution and with influential leaders external to the institution. Let others, particularly key administrators, know that your unit has a plan that advances programs, research, and service unique to your unit *and* that you have included initiatives consistent with the direction and priorities of the institution. Presidents and provosts value and showcase units that demonstrate initiative and commitment to institutional objectives. For example, it is not uncommon to hear presidents lament that their institution needs to be more responsive to undergraduate students, hoping that others within the institution will respond to this somewhat "fuzzy" request. This represents a golden opportunity for HPER units to include within their strategic plan some specific activities or directions that illustrate special efforts to serve undergraduate students (e.g., committing additional resources to advisement or developing special opportunities to engage undergraduates in research or outreach activities). Strategic plans help to convey that a HPER unit understands the importance of using its resources to further its specific mission as well as larger institutional priorities.

Quality Is Essential

An understanding of higher education issues, local institutional priorities, and strategic plans is important, but it is difficult to promote an HPER unit in a convincing manner unless the services offered by the unit are of high quality. The measures of quality will vary from institution to institution. However, some of the quality indicators that have been used frequently include: program size; the number of students served; professional accreditation and institutional reviews of undergraduate and graduate programs; productivity of faculty (e.g., number of published papers and books, professional presentations, and awards; amount of external funds secured); and demographics of students (e.g., gender; diversity; grade point average; awards; scores on tests such as the Scholastic Aptitude Test and the Graduate Record Exam; success in securing professional positions or admission to graduate school). The goal of an administrator is to aggregate these data such that the sum of the various parts become indicators of the unit's productivity, with trend lines identifying areas of excellence, growth, and needed improvement. In establishing and maintaining a viable set of quality indicators, it is important to rely, when possible, on data generated by other sources within the institution (e.g., the Office of Budget and Planning) or external to the institution (e.g., a published ranking of graduate programs).

While national and regional visibility is valuable in building a case for quality, it is essential that administrators also understand and value the culture within their institution. As Thomas (1998) observed, prominent programs within our field have been eliminated, but it is difficult to identify programs viewed as outstanding within their institution that have been eliminated. This suggests that internal program audits and reviews should be taken very seriously. Although many administrators fear institutional reviews of undergraduate and graduate programs and complain (rightfully so) of the amount of time and energy required to prepare for such reviews, the interaction with the review committee and this committee's final report provide an excellent means of showcasing a unit and its accomplishments. In many institutions, reviewers from other departments are used to assess the integrity of HPER programs. Meetings and interactions with these reviewers can be used to communicate and clarify program offerings and to address questions and misperceptions about the unit's focus and goals.

In many institutions, internal and external reviews are submitted to governing boards (e.g., boards of trustees or regents). Again, this provides a valuable opportunity to showcase the quality of your department or college. Upon receiving reviews, members of governing boards have been heard to make comments such as, "We had no idea you conducted research and ran programs on osteoporosis," or "You really are different from the athletic department." While comments such as these are disconcerting, it is best to accept them graciously and to use them as an opportunity to build new relationships by inviting board members to visit the unit and see its faculty and programs in action.

Avoid the Temptation to Over-Specialize

As part of the effort to legitimize the place of HPER in institutions of higher education, many administrators and faculty in HPER units have defined their role and focus far too narrowly. Examples of this include eliminating activity or outdoor recreation offerings and distancing ourselves from our traditional roots in the preparation of physical education and health teachers. The rationale for this is not without merit, of course. Early leaders such as Franklin Henry (1964) have been thoughtful and persuasive in distinguishing between a discipline (i.e., the study of a specific and unique body of knowledge) and a profession (i.e., what it is that you do with this body of knowledge). Some interpreted Henry to mean that HPER units did not need to be encumbered with teaching physical activity classes to general university students or with preparing future teachers. We began to focus all of our efforts toward changing "physical education" to "kinesiology" and "health education" to "health promotion," and adding "leisure" to "recreation." We became busy developing specialized laboratories, redefining graduate education, and transforming ourselves into smaller, more "academic" units.

None of this was detrimental; to the contrary, these efforts have served the field very well. The problem is that some units took this to an extreme, such that their focus became very narrow, leading to a preponderance of highly specialized courses and programs that served fewer students (Scanlan, 1998). HPER units—particularly those housed within colleges or schools of education—that chose to reduce or eliminate their commitment to teacher education were seen as being adrift from the mission of the college. This created confusion and, of course, vulnerability.

Clearly, however, there is also danger in becoming too broad and offering too many programs with too few resources. The key is balance, with the caveat that today's educational climate suggests strongly that units must use their resources efficiently and effectively to touch as many individuals as possible. A successful program is one that is fully integrated into several aspects of the institution (Dunn, 1998). An excellent example of this is the success experienced by Oregon State University's (OSU) College of Health and Human Performance during the tumultuous period of the 1980s, when many similar programs were undergoing significant reductions, mergers, or elimination. This college's success is largely attributable to its efforts in connecting to almost every aspect of the university. These efforts included: a required concepts course on health and fitness as part of the baccalaureate core; a very popular elective physical activity program; an intramural program with varied offerings; a faculty-staff fitness program with over 500 participants; community outreach programs for children with disabilities; and focused but comprehensive undergraduate and graduate programs (Maksud, 1998). The breadth and success of the college was such that students, faculty, staff, and the president of OSU had uniformly positive perceptions of the program. Simply put, so many on the OSU campus received valuable services from the unit that there was little question as to the unit's viability and centrality within the institution.

All institutions rely to a large extent on "good citizenry"—that is, on the volunteer efforts of faculty and staff. One of the most effective strategies for enhancing the perception of any unit is having faculty and administrators strategically positioned on committees and organizations that drive the institution. These include prestigious opportunities such as serving as the president of the faculty or academic senate and accepting appointments from the president or trustees to serve as the chair of a blue-ribbon committee. Fortunately, several HPER faculty from prestigious institutions such as Penn State University have served recently as president of their faculty senate. Face-to-face interaction with faculty from throughout the campus on issues central to the institution helps others acknowledge that HPER faculty are bright, creative, responsive, and—surprise of all surprises—similar to faculty within other disciplines. These efforts help to establish our credibility within the institution and to dispel unspoken assumptions (e.g., that the HPER unit is responsible solely for athletics or, worse yet, that it is a sub-unit within the athletic department) (Zauner, 1998). Leadership roles in the faculty senate or on strategic committees (e.g., for diversity, student retention, technology) create opportunities for faculty to interact with campus leaders and, in some instances, trustees and government leaders. On most campuses, the president of the academic senate is a member of the president's cabinet and attends all meetings of the university trustees. Participation at this level allows for personal interactions that are essential to establishing trust and building relationships.

Being a team player within the institution is the responsibility of everyone within a unit, including the dean, chair, faculty, staff, and students. If each individual contributes in some way, it should not be difficult to have a "strategic" presence in, and connection with, all facets of institutional activity. Committee service has the reciprocal benefit of feeding information into the HPER unit so that it is fully abreast of developments within the institution. This can help to identify early adjustments that the unit might take to ensure that its mission and strategic plan have currency.

Good "citizenry" also means displaying a willingness to cooperate with and support other units (e.g., sharing laboratory space; supporting another unit's request for a degree program; sharing a faculty member's expertise; participating in events hosted or sponsored by other units). The intent of such efforts is to establish a presence and to communicate in visible ways that HPER staff care about the institution and the members of

HPER Staff Must Be "Good Citizens"

its community. All too often, one hears stories of a department's unwillingness to cooperate or negotiate on sensitive institutional issues. A successful strategy for developing favorable perceptions is to have the HPER unit postured as reasonable and helpful to others within the institution and the state system (Dunn, 1998; Locke, 1998). Governing entities (legislators, regents, and trustees) place high priority on units that look for ways to support others. They see efforts to cooperate as support for their goals of streamlining the system, creating efficiencies, reducing duplication and costs, and serving the needs of students. Specific steps that HPER units might take toward cooperation include engaging sister institutions in collaborative efforts to differentiate programs and working with community colleges so that students can transition seamlessly to four-year institutions.

Hold a Party, Offer "Free" Services, and Sponsor Seminars

HPER administrators and faculty frequently lament, "Why don't they understand who we are and what we do?" This rhetorical question has been responded to, in part, with some of the advice offered throughout this chapter. The intent of this chapter is to encourage creative thinking about how to get decision-makers to sympathize with our environment. The suggestions and possibilities are endless, and the specifics of how best to proceed must be decided within the context of individual institutions. Some suggestions that have been successfully implemented by others include sponsoring a blood drive, conducting cholesterol screenings, offering a free health and fitness assessment, and providing a no- or low-cost graded exercise test for the president's cabinet, deans, and chairs (Maksud, 1998). Sponsoring free health fairs on campus (preferably) or in specific settings such as a state capital provide opportunities to: demonstrate knowledge and professional competence; respond to questions about health in general; address specific inquiries related to role clarification (e.g., "What is an exercise physiologist or certified health education specialist?"); meet (and thank) elected officials and their staff; and establish connections that can be helpful for future needs. For example, the College of Health at the University of Utah (UU) provides a fitness program for the governor and his staff. This is a strictly professional service with fees similar to those charged others who participate in a faculty-staff fitness program. This program has provided positive health outcomes for the governor and allowed HPER faculty to become better acquainted with him and with other key officials. As an expression of his appreciation, the governor invited selected HPER faculty and graduate students to his annual ball, where one faculty member who is an accomplished violist entertained him and his guests! Interactions such as these create long-lasting positive perceptions and consequences.

Related to the above is the value of inviting officials to visit programs sponsored by the HPER unit. For example, in conjunction with its physical activity program for children with disabilities, the UU College of Health held an annual open house for parents, school officials, university guests, and key legislators, particularly those interested in disability issues. The open house allowed us to communicate our commitment to individuals with disabilities, the expertise we offer to those individuals, the value of our program to UU students, and, most important, the benefits of the program for its participants.

Sponsoring an annual seminar with an invited speaker of note is another technique that can be used to showcase an HPER unit. Such seminars are most successful if they can be underwritten by a corporate entity or made possible through a gift or endowment. The ingredients of an effective seminar include an excellent speaker on a "hot" topic, a welcoming speech by the HPER administrator, formal introduction by a special guest (e.g., the provost or a key legislator), a well-developed and presented speech of 45 minutes or less, a question-and-answer session, and a reception with refreshments following the presentation. A poster advertising the presentation should be created, and a special letter of invitation should be sent to selected university officials, including trustees, government officials, legislators and their aides, alumni, and donors. A seminar provides an opportunity to share information on an exciting topic, and a closing reception is a good opportunity to build relationships. Those who are invited but cannot attend will appreciate the invitation and recognize that the HPER unit is alive and well and doing exciting things.

Informal opportunities to connect with university officials and legislators can also be used successfully to build relationships. Mike Maksud, former Dean at Oregon State University, was very successful in using his skill and interest in fishing and crabbing to "lure" key university officials and their families into special outings at Yaquina Bay and the Santiam River in Oregon. He cited the non-business nature of these outings as helpful in building relationships that were useful in later university-related discussions (Maksud, 1998). Others have found golf outings, running clubs, and community organizations to be important venues for connecting with key officials outside of the university environment.

One of the most compelling transformations occurring in higher education today is the renewed interest in connecting the academy to community needs and concerns. Examples of this include the emphasis placed on service-learning, where students learn and benefit as they connect with and address societal issues in action-oriented ways. Lawson (1998) refers to this as our social responsibility, arguing that HPER is well-suited to serve society as one of the "helping professions." If we are committed to ensuring our long-term viability, it is essential that we respond to local community needs. HPER units should be able to identify several opportunities for community outreach activities for students, given that there are so many community needs (e.g., the plight of the homeless and elderly; declines in the health and fitness of youths; the alarming division between the haves and have-nots in access to and delivery of health care; the plight of minority communities with regard to many health indicators; drug, alcohol, and tobacco use among youths; the spread of sexually transmitted diseases). The key is to integrate opportunities so that they benefit the students' academic and professional goals and respond appropriately to the needs of the community.

Connect with the Community

For example, one HPER department with which I am familiar has a partnership with several communities directed toward assisting local agencies and families in their quest to help at-risk youths avoid illicit drugs. The partnership is a combined effort between the university (represented by the HPER department), the state (which attracts funds from the federal government for the project), and local community leaders (including several mayors). While the expertise from the university is essential to the success of the project, efforts are directed toward empowering the communities so that the programs belong to them. Coordinated efforts such as these place the HPER unit in the enviable position of addressing real social issues and, in the process, gaining respect, friends, and recognition within and outside the institution. Similar successful outreach activities have been reported by others (e.g., Cheffers, 1997; Martinek, 1997; Martinek & Hellison, 1997).

The benefits associated with community-intervention programs are many. Valuable services are provided to communities, and university students are given the opportunity to hone their skills under the watchful eyes of master practitioners. If established correctly, these relationships enhance the quality of education for students and give them a much needed early introduction to the value of being of service to others. HPER units benefit from the interaction with community leaders and the opportunity to nurture these relationships into collaborative programs, including the potential for funded research. Most important, HPER administrators can point with pride to the community involvement of their faculty and students, and presidents and provosts can showcase the HPER unit as an example of a department or college that understands modern higher education and its responsibility to address social issues through partnerships with communities.

Summary

One of the major tasks facing HPER administrators is to help state officials, trustees, regents, presidents, and others within their institutions understand and appreciate HPER units and programs. As noted in this chapter, some in our field have suggested that the perception of key officials within and external to institutions may have accounted in part for the program reductions, eliminations, and mergers that have occurred with HPER units. This chapter has advanced several ideas that HPER administrators might employ to help create favorable perceptions of their unit. These suggestions include: encouraging HPER leaders to be cognizant of broad issues confronting higher education and of how these issues might affect their institution; developing a strategic plan congruent with the goals of their institution; avoiding the temptation to develop highly specialized, narrow programs; promoting the quality of their programs; being good institutional "citizens"; and promoting their unit through seminars, open houses, service, and special events. Implied throughout the chapter is the realization that what may be successful for one HPER unit may not work well within the culture of another unit or institution.

The good news is that HPER units and programs have a rich and proud history. Health, physical education, and recreation have contributed much to the betterment of society, and the programs and services provided by our units and by the professionals we prepare may be as highly valued today as at any time in our history. Administrators of HPER units would be wise to capture this current interest in their programs and to use the suggestions advanced in this chapter and other creative ideas to influence positively the perceptions that key leaders have of the role and future of HPER units in higher education.

John M. Dunn has served as an administrator in higher education for 20 years—as a department chair, assistant dean, associate provost, and dean. Professor Dunn has been widely recognized for his teaching, scholarship, and service, and he is a recipient of the NAPEHE Outstanding Administrator Award.

About the Author

References

Bouchard, C., Shephard, R. J., & Stephens, T. (Eds.). (1994). *Physical activity, fitness, and health.* Champaign, IL: Human Kinetics.

Cheffers, J. (1997). Tuesdays and Thursdays with Boston's inner-city youth. *Quest, 49,* 50-66.

Christina, R. W. (2000). Advancing engagement in kinesiology and physical education. *Quest, 52,* 315-329.

DePauw, K. P. (1998). Futuristic perspectives for kinesiology and physical education. *Quest, 50,* 1-8.

Dunn, J. M. (1998). Academic department survival: Lessons learned and future implications. *Quest, 50,* 179-184.

Dunn, J. M. (1999). Communicating with school boards: Position, power, and perseverance. *Quest, 51,* 157-163.

Ellis, M. J. (1998). Disasters on the west coast: Personal observations. *Quest, 50,* 121-125.

Franks, B. D. (1999). Good news: Altar call. *Quest, 51,* 194-199.

Henry, F. M. (1964). Physical education—An academic discipline. *Journal of Health, Physical Education & Recreation, 35,* 32, 33, 69.

Krahenbuhl, G. S. (1998). Higher education in the 21st century: The role of kinesiology and physical education. *Quest, 50,* 108-115.

Lawson, H. A. (1998). Here today, gone tomorrow? A framework for analyzing the development, transformation, and disappearance of helping fields. *Quest, 50,* 225-237.

Lawson, H. A. (1999). Education for social responsibility: Preconditions in retrospect and in prospect. *Quest, 51,* 116-149.

Locke, L. F. (1998). Advice, stories, and myths: The reactions of a cliffjumper. *Quest, 50,* 238-248.

Maksud, M. G. (1998). The Oregon State story: Strategy or happenstance? *Quest, 50,* 166-169.

Martinek, T. J. (1997). Serving underserved youth through physical activity. *Quest, 49,* 3-7.

Martinek, T. J., & Hellison, D. R. (1997). Fostering resiliency in underserved youth through physical activity. *Quest, 49,* 34-49.

Morgan, W. P. (1998). Restructuring departments: To merge or not to merge? *Quest, 50,* 134-148.

Morrow, J. R., Jr., & Blair, S. N. (1999). Promoting the Surgeon General's report on physical activity and health: Activities of the NCPPA. *Quest, 51,* 178-183.

Portch, S. (1999). The toughest teaching: Capturing attention, sketching pictures, and touching humanity. *Quest, 50,* 94-101.

San Jose State University. (2000). *Academic priorities planning process* [On-line]. Available: http://www.sjsu.edu/news_and_info/planning/workplan.html

Scanlan, T. K. (1998). Thriving versus surviving. *Quest, 50,* 126-133.

Singer, R. N. (1998). Gaining identity and respect for a department. *Quest, 50,* 149-158.

Thomas, J. R. (1998). Arizona State University: Prominence within the university is essential; Prominence within the academic field is nice. *Quest, 50,* 159-165.

U.S. Department of Health and Human Services. (1990). *Healthy people 2000: National health-promotion and disease-prevention objectives.* Washington, DC: U.S. Government Printing Office.

U.S. Department of Health and Human Services. (1996). *Physical activity and health—A report of the Surgeon General.* Atlanta, GA: Centers for Disease Control and Prevention.

Wilmore, J. H. (1998). Building strong academic programs for our future. *Quest, 50,* 103-107.

Zauner, C. W. (1998). Building a strong academic program at East Carolina University: Practical experiences. *Quest, 50,* 206-212.

2 The Changing Roles of Chairs and Deans

William J. Considine, *Dean, School of Health, Physical Education, and Recreation, Springfield College*

For every policy, procedure or process there is a rationale. Discover the rationale, examine the validity. If valid, initiate change.

○──┼──○ William J. Considine

When an individual makes the transition from being a faculty member to serving as chair or dean within a health, kinesiology, and/or leisure studies department, it seems that students, colleagues, and supervisors expect an instant metamorphosis. Suddenly, that individual is supposed to have all the answers, generate unlimited resources, be able to forecast the future (with extreme accuracy), and significantly influence the central administration—all this while maintaining the same collegial relationships as in the past. Unfortunately, as individuals grow into the role of chair or dean, their colleagues may perceive their personal relations to change. More likely, however, it is the role expectations that have changed, and these changes can in turn precipitate personal change. Like it or not, change will manifest itself in some form.

There are many popular sayings that reference change: "The only constant is change"; "The more things change, the more they stay the same"; "What goes around, comes around"; and so forth. Any individual who has been involved in higher-education administration in any capacity is likely convinced that the "stuff" that he or she deals with on a daily basis served as the original inspiration for such sayings.

Common Characteristics of Chairs and Deans

When discussing how the roles of chairs and deans are changing, one must remember that any attempts at describing and distinguishing these roles are, by necessity, generalizations. These roles are significantly influenced by factors such as: the size of the academic unit and institution in question; whether or not the institution is classified as a research university, extensive institution, or other type; and how individual chairs and deans choose to function.

15

Both deans and chairs are middle managers. Traditionally, chairs are faculty with some administrative responsibilities, while deans are administrators who represent academic and institutional interests and who may or may not be classified as faculty. Deans usually act as go-betweens for large, multi-departmental academic units and the central administration. Chairs usually represent a more singular unit composed of faculty charged with the responsibility of delivering a specific curriculum or program. Both deans and chairs are expected to understand, appreciate, and support the mission of the institution and to actualize it within their units. In most cases, a chair's responsibilities involve more direct support of the faculty, while a dean's advocacy for faculty is more indirect. The chair is more of a front-line faculty leader and representative with a greater managerial role.

Chairpersons "are neither pure faculty members nor regular administrators and yet are expected somehow to represent both sets of interests" (Bennett, 1982, p. 54). A dean, however, is more of a representative of the central administration, with the expectation that the will of this administration is to prevail; the task, then, is to convince the chair to make it happen. As Hecht, Higgerson, Gmelch, and Tucker (1999) put it, "Deans work 'in the middle ground' between the central administration that leads and coordinates the mission and direction of the institution and the department chairs who orchestrate the daily activities that make that mission manifest" (p. 197).

Both deans and chairs have multiple roles and tasks. Chairs are equally engaged in both planning and implementation, while deans are more likely to be engaged in planning than in direct implementation. A chair is a leader, scholar, teacher, manager, and colleague. A dean is a leader, a facilitator, and an advocate for both the school/college and the institution. A dean has ultimate—but less direct—responsibility for curriculum, whereas a chair has a significant and direct responsibility for it. The majority of a chair's efforts are directed internally in support of the students and the faculty within an academic unit. A dean's efforts may be more equally distributed between the larger academic unit, the institution, and external affairs: "The dean's primary role is to nurture relationships that involve others in making decisions, determining goals and objectives, and designing and implementing policies and programs" (Austin, Ahearn, & English, 1997, p. 3). A chair's primary role is to facilitate the delivery of high-quality instruction and to promote scholarship and service. There is little doubt that the chair is the point of contact through which implementation almost always flows. While there are many moments when chairs might feel underappreciated, most in higher education recognize their importance. "An institution can run for a long time with an inept president, but not for long with an inept chairperson," stated J. W. Peltason, past president of the American Council on Education (Tucker, 1984, p. xi).

Expectations are changing for both chairs and deans. The notions of accountability and "doing more with less" have significantly influenced the roles of both. Chairs are being pulled more into the role of administrators with some faculty responsibilities. Deans are also being pulled further along toward institutional administration. While development activities have been assigned to deans for some time now, this role is beginning to manifest itself at the chair level as well. Chairs are moving more toward implementing institutional goals and priorities, albeit through their individual departments.

In his recent research, Yam (1999) reported that physical education and kinesiology chairpersons derived more satisfaction from responsibilities centered on students and research activities, and less satisfaction from those associated with documenting, budgeting, and managing staff. Unfortunately, chairing a department today leaves less and less time for students and research and demands more and more time for the latter activities. Yam (1999) also found that;

> *sources of the negative feelings such as frustration, irritation, disappointment, stress, aggravation, and being overwhelmed came from being the middle administrator, work overload, personnel problems, and role conflicts of being teacher/chairperson or researcher/chairperson...positive feelings included satisfaction, reward, enjoyment, and fulfillment often linked to either personal or departmental accomplishment. (pp. 49-50)*

Deans likely have similar feelings regarding their roles and responsibilities.

Discussion of chairing most academic departments can be generic, since there are many duties and expectations common to that role. However, there can be a wide variation of responsibilities for chairs and deans of health, physical education, kinesiology, and/or leisure studies departments, depending on the programs housed within the academic unit and the unit structure itself. Typically, chairs of kinesiology and physical education departments are responsible for coordinating facility use with athletics and intramural programs. Shared personnel between the athletics program and the academic unit may also create unique responsibilities for both the chair and the dean. The administration of a "skills" program usually generates added responsibilities such as: selecting and assigning graduate assistants; hiring adjuncts; contracting for services; managing course fees and equipment rentals; providing transportation; and ensuring risk management. A health-program administrator may inherit responsibilities for facilitating certification qualification. Leisure-services departments are often affiliated with outdoor facilities and operations such as camps, adventure activities, and extended travel arrangements for student groups. The norms for an administrator of health, physical education, kinesiology, and/or leisure services are quite different from those encountered by administrators of "traditional" academic units.

Chairs and Deans in HPER

In preparation for writing this chapter, the author conducted an informal survey among his administrative colleagues (members of the college and university administrator's council), asking them to rank the changes that have occurred in various organizational and personal factors related to their administrative duties. The results showed some wide variability, but some centrality as well. As with any survey, the results were influenced by the circumstances of each individual and the organizational climate of the institution; therefore, no scientific claims will be made about validity. Rather, the results will be presented to reflect the perceptions of the respondents, with the hope that some insight and comfort might be provided to those entering the world of higher education administration.

Changing Roles: A Survey

As one might anticipate, personnel-related tasks such as hiring, retention, tenure, promotion, and evaluation were perceived as having undergone significant change of late. As described in the literature, these tasks have become more detailed, require more documentation, and demand more time and attention than in the past. In past decades, chairs were not confronted with extensive employment regulations, detailed documentation procedures, or such involved assessment processes. Further, it has become more difficult to match faculty expertise to program needs. As faculty become more specialized, the task of redirecting or initiating programs and courses becomes all the more challenging. The respondents also suggested that faculty commitment has changed. Perhaps a shift from a balance of departmental and personal goals to a more pronounced career-achievement paradigm is beginning to emerge.

The task of defining and conveying faculty duties was ranked and listed as having undergone a moderate amount of change, but other factors such as grievances, termination proceedings, personnel files, professional ethics, adjuncts, and compensation were ranked lower, indicating that they had undergone less change over the years.

All of these perceptions would seem to suggest that personnel-related issues demand a significant portion of an administrator's attention and time. In fact, some of the experienced administrators in this survey indicated that they now spend 70 to 80 percent of their time on such issues. Obviously, that leaves little time for all of their other duties. No wonder the workload for those with administrative responsibilities is escalating!

Keeping up with technology also appears to be a continuing challenge. Since technology itself changes so rapidly, the tasks of acquiring and maintaining adequate equipment have become increasingly challenging for administrators. According to the respondents, staying on the cutting edge of technology seems less of a problem than assuring the availability of functional equipment.

Program delivery was rated moderately high in the survey. The curricular approval/revision process seems to have undergone some changes. Based upon observation, curricular change requires more paperwork, more approval signatures, and more time from both the initiating faculty member and the department chair. External accreditation standards, along with initiatives such as outcomes assessment, strategic planning, and program review, impose further demands on department personnel.

Although budgeting was not rated high compared to personnel issues, technology, or program delivery, several interesting insights can be gleaned from the subcategories of this organizational factor. For example, it is evident that certain recent institutional changes in the budgeting process had already been experienced by the respondents: that is, administrators may find that a supposedly "new" approach or procedure is simply a slightly modified version of a previous form. Although the institutional approach to budgeting may have changed, it doesn't seem to have affected the respondents as much as the level of funding has. As one would expect, trying to figure out how to make allocations match extended needs is an ever-present challenge, while preparing and submitting the budget requests, no matter what their form, is a task that simply "gets done."

Based on the rankings within the category of organizational structure, it seems that some institutions have undergone significant "restructuring" while others have experienced little structural change. Any administrator who has experienced reconfiguration of academic units at an institution appreciates the time and energy that is involved in the planning and implementation of such "realignment." And anyone who stays in an administrative capacity for a considerable length of time is sure to be involved in some form of reorganization. Higher education seems to have a penchant for reinventing itself. For those who have gone through such a change, it remains a memorable event.

Facility use was ranked seventh out of the nine organizational factors. Maintenance of facilities was ranked slightly higher than scheduling classes and events in the facilities. Although there was no indicator of such, it may be assumed that this perception of slightly greater change in the former area was not caused by an increase in the quality or quantity of maintenance!

Although much administrative attention is focused on internal policies and procedures, these seem to have undergone less change than personnel-related factors. The tasks of formulating, implementing, and complying with policies and procedures have not changed a great deal. Perhaps that is because there has always been a preponderance of policies and procedures in higher education. Legal issues and human-resources processes were the highest ranked tasks within the policies and procedures category. With the increase in civil litigation in society in general, it is logical that administrative involvement in legal issues has increased as well.

Public relations and fundraising were the two lowest ranked factors. Although there are administrative duties involving both internal and external public relations, these functions were not perceived to have undergone significant change. This perception is influenced by the fact that the majority of the respondents were chairs rather than deans. Although most chairs have yet to be drawn into the full complexities of public affairs and fundraising, indications are that they will be called upon to do so in the near future.

Regarding those factors with a direct, personal impact on them, the respondents ranked their assigned tasks as having undergone the most change. This would suggest that both the nature and quantity of what administrators are expected to do has changed. The greater number of duties combined with the intricacies of prescribed processes have increased the time that it takes to complete assigned tasks.

Self-initiated tasks were ranked second within this category, slightly ahead of administrative control. The commitment levels of faculty, the quality of students, and the commitment levels of students were next in ranking, although there was a marked difference in the strength of the rankings, as the former two factors received much more of a consensus than the latter. There is a perception that the commitment level of faculty has changed over the years—that they are less likely to extend themselves for the welfare of the academic unit than they were in the past. Furthermore, much has been written about the declining preparedness of students entering college, and now it seems that administrators sense a decline in student commitment to the act of learning as well. Other personal factors such as support, recognition, rewards, efficiency, and satisfaction were ranked low. This would suggest that these factors have undergone little change, or that they are minimally important to the respondents.

While the results of this informal survey do not reveal any startling discoveries, the reported perceptions of these experienced administrators do indicate where change has demanded their extra attention and energy. Twenty years ago, HPER chairs and deans did not have to confront challenges such as outcomes assessment, enrollment management, electronically generated degree competition, software licensing, or the extensive generation of outside funding. Furthermore, the form and degree of accountability have changed, personnel-related responsibilities and processes have become more sophisticated, external influence by governing or accrediting bodies has increased, and the expectations of all constituencies for leadership and management have both diversified and escalated.

While issues such as these will affect the activities of deans and chairs, none will most likely displace personnel issues as the factor commanding most of their time and attention. Continuous change is a given and will certainly test new and aspiring administrators. However, it is the contention of this author that getting faculty to fulfill all of their responsibilities at a level of excellence will remain the foremost challenge of any administrator. After all, we must not forget that academic units are really people.

About the Author

William J. Considine is entering his 25th year as an administrator at Springfield College, currently serving as Dean of the School of Health, Physical Education, and Recreation.

References

Austin, M. J., Ahearn, F. L., & English, R. A. (Eds.). (1997). *The professional school dean: Meeting the leadership challenges.* San Francisco: Jossey-Bass.

Bennett, J. (1982). Ambiguity and abrupt transition in the department chairperson's role. *Educational Record, 63*(4), 53-56.

Hecht, I. W. D., Higgerson, M. L., Gmelch, W. H., & Tucker, A. (1999). *The department chair as academic leader.* Phoenix, AZ: Oryx.

Tucker, A. (1984). *Chairing the academic department: Leadership among peers* (2nd ed.). New York: Macmillan.

Yam, R. H. M. (1999). *Understanding the experiences of physical education department chairpersons: A phenomenological interviewing study.* Unpublished doctoral dissertation, Springfield College, Springfield, MA.

3 Expectations and Responsibilities within Administrative Support Roles

Jan Rintala, *Professor and Assistant Chair, Department of Kinesiology and Physical Education, Northern Illinois University*

Some days you step in it . . . some days you don't.

Jan Rintala

As with any complex enterprise, a college, school, or department within an institution of higher education cannot succeed based solely on the leadership skills and talents of one individual. The purpose of this chapter is to highlight those persons other than department chairs and deans who carry out necessary administrative responsibilities.

The challenges in writing on such a topic are many. First, while there is a substantial body of literature related to the roles of chairs and deans, there is a dearth of information addressing administrative support roles. For this reason, much of the information in this chapter is inferred from the literature on chairs and deans or based on the professional experiences of the author.

A second challenge emerges because of the great variability among health, kinesiology, and leisure-studies units. Many different parameters determine the structure of such units: for example, the size of the unit; the number of disciplines and program areas represented; the levels of degree programs; and the relative importance of teaching, scholarship, artistry, and service. While all of these factors influence the role of the chair or the dean, there is still a common core of responsibilities that each must fulfill, regardless of other variables. These responsibilities include serving as faculty developers, managers, leaders, and scholars (Gmelch & Miskin, 1993). As will become evident shortly, however, no similar core of responsibilities exists for those who serve in administrative support roles.

This chapter will look at (1) the ways in which administrative support roles can increase a unit's effectiveness, (2) the reasons a faculty member may have for assuming one of these roles, and (3) important logistical concerns such as load adjustment and compensation issues. The points raised

21

here are intended to help academic units consider whether the way in which they are currently accomplishing administrative tasks might be improved by some altering of responsibilities or structure. They can also help chairs and deans in the selection or recruitment of people into these roles. For those who may find themselves moving into these roles (by choice or default), this chapter may assist them in their transition.

The remainder of the chapter is written primarily from the perspective of departments. This is done partly for ease of reading, but also because it is assumed that the level at which the greatest variability of issues exists is the departmental level. The roles of associate and assistant deans are likely to be more clearly delineated at this level than are the many different support roles. Administrative support roles at the college level are also more likely to be full-time positions, so some of the issues related to work load, compensation, and negotiating multiple roles are less relevant. Certain portions of what follows are relevant to each academic level, though. As one reads this chapter, it will be important to carefully consider which of the points raised are applicable to one's own unique situation.

Importance of Administrative Support Roles

There are both practical and philosophical reasons for chairs to have assistance with the administrative duties of their department. At perhaps the most basic level of practicality, there may simply be more administrative duties than one individual can humanly handle. Even in departments where it was once reasonable for one person to do it all, this may no longer be true today. Some ongoing tasks may require more time and effort than they once did. For example, faculty recruitment and retention are more time-consuming than ever, especially as departments strive to attain and maintain a diverse faculty. This diversity may require the chair to devote more attention to facilitating a department culture in which all faculty feel valued.

The writing of reports and program reviews has also become more labor-intensive. As the standards of accrediting bodies change and new accrediting bodies emerge, and as departments add new programs that require accreditation, chairs may find themselves within several different accreditation cycles at any given time. Some of these accrediting bodies include the National Council for Accreditation of Teacher Education (NCATE), the Commission on the Accreditation of Allied Health Education Programs (CAAHEP), and the North American Society for Sport Management (NASSM). This difficulty is further compounded by demands for accountability from the university, state boards of higher education, and legislative bodies.

There are also responsibilities that may not have previously been a major part of a chair's job, but that are now finding their way into the regular expectations for the position. One of these is student recruitment and retention; as with faculty, there are issues of diversity here, not only in terms of race and gender, but also in terms of students who are non-traditional in a variety of ways. Furthermore, as legislatures decrease the percentage of a public institution's budget that they will continue to support, seeking external funds for scholarships, facilities expansion, or large equipment purchases may now become a bigger role for chairs in such institutions. These are but a few examples, but assuming that the other duties of chairs have not disappeared, something must be delegated if previously minor demands are increased.

Another very practical reason for delegating certain administrative tasks to others is to attract effective individuals to chair positions and keep them there. One of the drawbacks for many faculty who might consider serving as a chair is the resultant sacrifice of some of their pedagogical, scholarly, and artistic commitments. Restructuring the responsibilities of chairs and redistributing some of their tasks may increase the willingness of some faculty to take on the position and stay in it. Enabling chairs to retain their involvement in teaching, scholarship, and artistry also benefits both the department and the profession.

If individuals in support roles routinely handle specific administrative assignments, the chair may be able to perform the remaining tasks more effectively. One of the challenges for chairs is to avoid falling into what Gmelch, Miskin, and Seedorf (1996) call "an endless activity trap" (p. 3). They suggest that it is important for chairs to focus on high-payoff (HIPO) tasks and delegate (if they cannot eliminate) low-payoff (LOPO) tasks. Two items they identify as LOPO tasks are excessive committee work and "administrivia." There may be many activities that could easily be completed by others without compromising the ultimate responsibility of the chair for the operation of the department. Preliminary work on scheduling, curricular revisions, reports, placement of student teachers and interns, and equipment purchases, to name a few, could all be performed by others. Once this preliminary work is done—often by those who are involved more directly with the issue at hand in the first place—the chair can enter the various processes at key decision-making points.

Beyond these very practical reasons for having others assist the chair with administrative activities, there may also be philosophical justifications. One of the most basic is a commitment to a less hierarchical department structure (Gmelch & Miskin, 1993). There may be several advantages to this approach to departmental functioning and decision-making. One is that it enables the department to more fully utilize the strengths—and minimize the weaknesses—of all staff members. No one individual will be equally effective at all tasks. If there are others in the department who can complete some jobs with even greater effectiveness than the chair, then the department as a whole stands to gain from delegation.

One of the challenges in a hierarchical structure is that individuals tend to focus on their own domain and fail to see the larger picture. They become unconcerned about the whole because "that's the chair's job." This may even lead to an unwillingness to work towards the good of the whole. Having several members of the faculty serve in administrative support roles may mitigate this problem. Administrative tasks require that one consider multiple factors and perspectives. When faculty have the opportunity (or responsibility) for such tasks, they may exhibit a willingness and ability to see beyond their own classes or research agendas. Furthermore, as they interact with others while fulfilling their administrative responsibilities, they may gain a knowledge of and a sensitivity to other faculty members and programmatic concerns.

The presence of other faculty in leadership positions may also contribute to a sense of personal investment on the part of the faculty as a whole, since they will see that they are able to influence the direction of the department more directly. Those faculty who have specific programmatic responsibilities (e.g., graduate director, director of teacher education, director of an exercise science program) may also serve on a departmental advisory committee, just as chairs may serve on an advisory committee to their dean. Because of their daily involvement with programmatic aspects of the department, these individuals can provide input on facility and equipment needs or assist in the development of position descriptions for new or replacement faculty. These new positions may be able to cut across programmatic areas and meet multiple needs based on the discussions of an advisory committee.

While having a greater number of people involved in tasks and decision-making may not always be the most time-efficient method of operation, those who believe in a more participative department culture will assert that it is a better way for the department to carry out its mission. The chair benefits by having the opportunity to hear ideas and approaches that she or he may not have considered, and if those in administrative support roles function as an advisory committee, ideas may emerge through discussion that no single individual would have developed on his or her own.

Kinds of Administrative Support Roles

So, just what are some of these administrative support roles? Many tasks may be performed by others without there being a specific title affiliated with the role. Some of these activities include scheduling, coordinating registration efforts, working with various university offices on student recruitment and orientation, and working with community colleges to ensure a smoother transition for transfer students. However, in reflecting on my own knowledge of departmental structures and examining various departmental web pages, I have found that many administrative support roles have established titles:

- assistant chairs
- program directors (e.g., graduate, undergraduate, health education, teacher education, exercise science, sport management, athletic training, recreation, dance, aquatics, basic instruction)
- directors of centers (research centers or institutes)
- coordinators (of advising, student teaching, internships, student organizations, scholarship programs, facilities, technology)
- laboratory directors
- directors of outreach programs (faculty/staff exercise and wellness, community fitness, community dance, motor-skill development for community youths)
- coordinators for international study
- directors of off-campus programs

The types of support roles, as well as the specific responsibilities for each of these positions, will obviously vary according to the unique programmatic concerns and mission of each department, but it is evident that there are many ways in which faculty can become involved in administrative responsibilities.

Reasons for Serving in Support Roles

The existence of administrative support roles is basically moot if there are no people willing to step into those roles. There are several important reasons for pursuing such positions. One of these reasons was alluded to earlier, in the discussion of personal investment: that is, faculty may wish to have a more active role or voice in shaping the direction of their department. Another reason is that a faculty member may be contemplating a career move into an administrative position (e.g., chair), and one of these assistant, director, or coordinator positions is a logical first step. According to Hecht, Higgerson, Gmelch, and Tucker (1999), one of the challenges facing new chairs is that they have little, if any, previous administrative experience. Support roles provide an important learning opportunity that can ameliorate some of this lack of experience if the individual should later move into a chair position. This also gives faculty members a risk-free means of determining whether a more involved administrative role is really what they want.

Other people simply like the variety and the challenge of the chair position. While some faculty members would prefer that there be little change in their day-to-day activities—even to the point of resisting changes in their teaching schedules or the rooms in which they teach—others need periodic change and new challenges. An opportunity to assume one of these leadership roles may provide that needed change and give faculty members a chance to use some skills that their regular faculty assignments may not require.

In some departments, administrative roles are viewed as part of the service component of faculty responsibilities, and faculty members simply accept that taking their turn in these roles is an expectation. Some of these positions may be filled on a rotational basis, in a manner similar to that in which some departments fill the position of chair. Finally, there may be economic reasons motivating a faculty member to assume one of these positions, since they may include a stipend or employment during summers and between sessions.

Logistical and Transitional Concerns

When a need or opportunity exists for an administrative support role to be created or filled, there are several logistical and transitional concerns that should be addressed before any final decisions are made by the chair or the individual considering the position. One of the first steps is to be certain that the specific responsibilities of the position are clearly delineated. It is important to have a list of these responsibilities; while it is impossible to list every task, all parties should know the expectations to the greatest extent possible. The position description and responsibilities may also need to be revised periodically. This can be done as part of an annual meeting between the chair and the administrative support person when they review the past year and discuss plans for the future. It is also important for a description of the responsibilities of all administrative positions to be available to all members of the department. These descriptions can be included in the department handbook so that all members know to whom they should go for certain questions or concerns.

Another very important issue is workload. There is an increasing tendency among faculty today to be unwilling to simply take on additional tasks without having adjustments made to their other responsibilities. If the administrative responsibilities require a significant amount of time, then teaching or research expectations may be modified. Decisions need to be made carefully, not only so that the faculty member involved has a reasonable opportunity to successfully handle all of his or her responsibilities, but also to lessen dissension and resentment among other members of the faculty. In many departments, there are certain faculty members who are quite concerned about how much work everyone is doing. If they perceive that too much load adjustment is being given, internal morale problems can arise. If an insufficient workload adjustment is given, however, support persons may not satisfactorily complete their duties or may simply give up their administrative roles "because it just isn't worth it." In many institutions, it is also necessary to be very clear about workload because of reporting and accountability processes set up by governing boards and state agencies.

In some units, it may not be possible to make adjustments in other responsibilities: the classes simply must be taught. It is also possible that giving up any part of such responsibilities is not what the faculty member desires. In these cases, there may be other ways to compensate the person for assuming additional administrative responsibilities. One such way is to pay an administrative stipend. If the person must perform duties between sessions or be available at least part-time during the summer, then a salary adjustment for that period of time may be acceptable.

Budget constraints or university policy may prohibit direct monetary compensation, but there are other ways in which a faculty member can be compensated. Being offered administrative support duties may, in fact, be one of the few situations in which a returning faculty member is in a position to negotiate. The negotiations are limited only by institutional regulations and by the creativity of those involved. Faculty may consider adjusting their teaching schedules, perhaps to clear larger blocks of time for administrative tasks. For example, one may teach the same number of hours per term, but teach fewer preps over the course of the year.

If faculty are involved in teaching at off-campus sites, this may also be an item to consider during negotiations. Factors such as proximity to home or extra compensation may make it appealing for an administrative support person to teach off-campus. Or, if teaching off-campus is a departmental expectation that the person would prefer to avoid, this could be an item of negotiation as well. In our college, assistant chairs are on a full-time administrative appointment. Full-time administrators who choose to teach are not eligible for compensation if the course is taught on-campus. The chair or assistant chair may, however, teach a course at one of the off-campus sites for extra compensation.

There may be little flexibility in the personnel line item of the budget, but the chair may have some latitude with other line items. Travel support could be increased, or additional equipment (e.g., new or upgraded technology components) could be purchased to enhance the individual's teaching, research, or artistic activities. Perhaps a graduate-student administrative or research assistant could be provided.

Another very important concern centers on how the person's administrative tasks are incorporated into personnel evaluation procedures, especially tenure, promotion, and merit evaluations. It is important not only for the individual to know these things, but also that they be known by all who will be involved in the evaluation process, including department and college personnel committees. The way in which the administrative assignment is to be weighted in any overall evaluation must be established beforehand (e.g., as 15 percent of a final merit rating), and procedures for assessing administrative performance must be laid out as well. This can create challenges because administrative tasks are not encompassed within the typical personnel evaluation information (e.g., student evaluations, peer observations of teaching, teaching portfolios, and documentation of research and service activities).

With some administrative roles, it may be possible to gather evaluative feedback from those in a position to provide relevant information. For example, if one wishes to evaluate a graduate program director, a form with forced-choice questions and opportunities for open-ended responses can be given to members of the graduate faculty and a sample of graduate students. These persons may not be in a position to answer all questions, but there may be sufficient information to provide some basis for evaluation. In some cases, the number of people who would be in a position to respond might be so small that either anonymity could not be assured or factors unrelated to performance would taint the usefulness of the response. In still other instances, the only person in a position to evaluate is the person actually doing the job; thus self-reporting or self-evaluation may be the only source of information.

As a final note here, if administrative service is not taken into account or valued during the tenure process, non-tenured faculty may want to delay taking on these roles until after tenure has been secured. The ways in which such service affects promotion may be less critical, but it is only fair to the faculty member that she or he understands these effects from the onset. Having this discussion with each faculty member is part of the developmental responsibilities of the chair.

For those units in which the faculty are members of a collective-bargaining unit, many of the above issues may be moot. The collective-bargaining agreement may already stipulate the selection process, responsibilities, workload adjustments, compensation issues, and evaluative procedures for administrative support persons.

Once a faculty member has assumed an administrative support position, he or she will need to learn the various new skills that the position entails. Given their faculty-development role, chairs may be involved in helping new assistants in this learning.

Faculty-Development Concerns

As with any new position, one must quickly learn about the new forms and reports that need to be completed. There may also be new reporting lines, and new committees and individuals across campus with whom one needs to establish working relationships. These transitions, while occasionally time-consuming, resemble the kinds of transitional processes faculty will have undergone throughout their professional lives.

There are other adjustments, however, that will be novel because the transition involves moving into an administrative capacity. Many of these will be the same adjustments that the chair had to make, and chairs who are willing to recall their own transitions are in a better position to assist these new administrators. One common challenge is balancing the roles of administrator, teacher, and scholar. It is very easy for an administrative position to take up much more of one's time and energy than the workload adjustment may provide. It is important for the individual to find ways of maintaining balance and developing work strategies that work best for him or her.

One must also adjust to a decrease in autonomy. As a faculty member, one is basically responsible for oneself and one's students. Faculty teach classes, hold office hours, and attend committee meetings: beyond that, their time is theirs to control. As faculty move into administrative positions, they become accountable to others as well, and the flexibility of their schedules may be more restricted. This can be particularly problematic when the majority of their responsibilities still lie within the traditional faculty role.

Faculty also assume a different position in relation to the institutional bureaucracy once they take on administrative duties. For many faculty, bureaucracy is something either to ignore (seen as the responsibility of the chair and other administrators) or to react against (seen as that which puts up barriers or creates unnecessary work). Depending on the new administrative assignment, one is now in a position of needing to understand the bureaucracy, become effective within it, and perhaps even defend it to one's colleagues.

Change can also occur in some aspects of a new administrator's relationships with colleagues. As a faculty member comes to be seen as an administrator, people may become more guarded in their conversations with him or her. It is also possible that faculty will use new administrators—especially those in assistant or program-director roles—as a conduit to the chair. This can be an important role, as chairs and deans need people on whom they can rely to report to them with important issues that are occurring within the department or college. There is a need for someone who can go to the chair or dean and tell them when something isn't working—even if that something is the administrator's pet project.

In serving as a conduit, it becomes very important to determine when one listens to information without acting on it, when one takes the information to the chair, and when one indicates to the faculty member that she or he needs to take the matter directly to the chair. There are many situations in which one should not serve as a conduit, such as conflicts among faculty and staff. It may be important that the administrative support person listen to complainants and perhaps provide some suggestions for how they might want to proceed (one would do this much for any colleague), but conflicts between faculty need to be worked out by the individuals or taken directly to the chair. It is important to clarify with the chair the preferred procedures for such situations.

The chair should also clarify those items over which support personnel have autonomy and those matters that should be shared with the chair before proceeding. The chair is ultimately responsible for the administrative activities of the department; while there are many routine items that can be completed by those in support positions without the chair's oversight, there are other items that the chair may wish to see first (e.g., items that go to persons external to the department or that convey a departmental stance). There may be a transitional process here as well. The chair may wish to look at some items the first time or two around and then indicate that the support person can just proceed on similar items in the future. It is important to develop a balance. Faculty are selected for these positions because it is assumed that they can do administrative work. The chair must feel confident that the jobs are being done, and the support person must have some autonomy in the position. Again, one of the primary reasons for having these positions is because the chair has plenty to do already. If everything requires the chair's approval, or if the support person is uncomfortable moving forward without such approval, then this purpose is defeated. Communication and continued negotiation about these issues are important.

Finally, when faculty serve in administrative roles, they need to see a more global department, college, and university picture that goes beyond their own disciplinary perspectives and concerns. There are many advantages to having faculty who are able to do this. However, the chair may have to assist new administrators in becoming aware of these alternative ways of seeing things.

Summary

The items above are by no means an exhaustive discussion of administrative support roles in health, kinesiology, and leisure-studies units. To reiterate a point made early in the chapter, there are many unique characteristics of individual departments, colleges, and faculty members that will influence the organizational structures and the distribution of responsibilities. There are other models that could be considered (e.g., hiring people without faculty rank for some administrative tasks, such as coordinating advisement, student recruitment, facilities, and technology). Units should periodically assess whether there have been changes in their focus, personnel, resources, or programs that may suggest new configurations and assignments. There may be a tendency to simply maintain department administrative structures without considering whether those structures are still productive. This assessment may be a part of an ongoing strategic planning process or may emerge during times of transition (e.g., a turnover of personnel). There are always challenges in delegating administrative responsibilities, finding the right people to assume these responsibilities, and helping these people learn new skills and roles. The payoffs for both the individuals and the academic unit as a whole, however, make these administrative support positions well worth the challenge.

Acknowledgment

The author wishes to thank George White, a dean at Montana State University–Billings, for his willingness to provide editorial feedback on this article.

About the Author

Jan Rintala is a professor and assistant chair in the Department of Kinesiology and Physical Education at Northern Illinois University. She has served as assistant chair or assistant to the chair for four years.

References

Gmelch, W. H., & Miskin, V. D. (1993). *Leadership skills for department chairs.* Boston: Anker.

Gmelch, W. H., Miskin, V. D., & Seedorf, R. G. (1996). The journey of the department chair. *Newsletter of the Center for the Study of the Department Chair, 5*(2), 1-4.

Hecht, I. W. D., Higgerson, M. L., Gmelch, W. H., & Tucker, A. (1999). *The department chair as academic leader.* Phoenix, AZ: Oryx.

4 Surviving in Higher Education: Knowledge and Action Are the Keys

Jerry R. Thomas, *Professor and Chair, Department of Health and Human Performance, Iowa State University*

Additional problems are the offspring of poor solutions.
— Mark Twain as quoted by Jerry R. Thomas

Our field is changing along with the rest of higher education; if we hope to survive, we need to plan for change. Below is a list of selected kinesiology programs—many at highly visible research institutions—that have changed drastically in the past 20 to 30 years, most of them involuntarily.

Eliminated/Downsized	Remained Strong/Strengthened[1]
Florida State University	Arizona State University
University of Arizona	Indiana University
University of California at Berkeley	Iowa State University
University of California at Los Angeles	Oregon State University
University of Iowa	Texas A&M University
University of Missouri	University of Florida
University of Oregon	University of Georgia
University of Southern California	University of Maryland
University of Washington	University of North Carolina at
Washington State University	Greensboro

What have the strong departments done differently from those that have been eliminated or downsized? To answer that question, consideration must be given to the environment outside of higher education as well as to internal factors.

First and foremost, American society has changed in ways that have forced a response from colleges and universities. Higher education is no longer an elitist activity—that changed with the end of World War II and the introduction of the GI Bill. Furthermore, parents want a better life for their children, and higher education is a means to obtain such a life—for

31

one thing, college graduates have higher average salaries than high school graduates. There will be an increase in the number of college students in the near future, but a larger proportion of these students will come from the poorer and less-educated sectors of our society (Almanac, 1999). As noted by Krahenbuhl (1998), "the number of high-achieving, parent-financed, straight-out-of-high-school, full-time, residential college students will change little or perhaps decline" (p. 109). In addition, many more adult students will be entering (or re-entering) colleges and universities to enhance their standard of living and enjoyment of life.

Internal and External Factors in Department Survival

In addition to these demographic changes in colleges and universities since the late 1940s, other external factors are having major impacts on higher education, including: the Carnegie Foundation for the Advancement of Teaching's plan for expanding the categories of higher-education institutions from "research," "doctoral," "comprehensive," and "liberal arts" to those listed in figure 4.1; and new federal, private, and foundation funding for programs and research (e.g., from the National Institutes of Health, National Science Foundation, U.S. Department of Agriculture, Department of Energy, Danforth Foundation, Rockefeller Foundation, Ford Foundation). In addition, colleges and universities are rated on any number of factors including program quality, research and development expenditures, fundraising, endowments, and the number of National Merit Scholars they recruit. Colleges and universities also strive to be accredited by regional accreditation groups (e.g., North Central, Southern) and/or specialized accrediting groups (e.g., for education, the National Council for the Accreditation of Teacher Education; for athletic training, the Commission on Allied Health Education Programs). Furthermore, most colleges and universities are finding reductions in state support for higher education, as entitlement programs (e.g., health care, public schools, prisons, roads) compete for state funding.

Internal factors also play a role in what a department does and how it plans. For example, one must consider where a department is located—within a health-related college (e.g., allied health), a college of liberal arts and sciences, a college of education, or a stand-alone college (e.g., of health and human performance). This determines the institution's view of the department and, sometimes, the department's name. Departments in colleges of liberal arts and sciences are likely to place substantial value on external funding, and on preparing students with broad backgrounds in science and humanities, and less emphasis on preparing students for jobs. Departments in colleges of education typically find that they need to establish their role in preparing teachers, an area attracting much less student interest than in the past.

Many of our departments have attracted large numbers of undergraduate majors because of widespread interest in health, sport, exercise, physical activity, and leisure. Yet few of these individuals choose the traditional model of preparing to be health and/or physical education teachers. Most are interested in the fitness industry, athletic training, community health, parks and recreation, sports medicine, or sport management.

Doctoral/Research Universities (Extensive)
❖ confer at least 50 doctorates per year in 15 or more disciplines—3.8% of all institutions

Doctoral/Research Universities (Intensive)
❖ at least 10 doctorates per year in 3 or more disciplines—2.9%

Master's Colleges and Universities (Comprehensive I)
❖ range of programs through the master's, with at least 40 master's degrees annually—12.7%

Master's Colleges & Universities (Comprehensive II)
❖ range of programs through the master's, with at least 20 master's degrees annually—3.3%

Baccalaureate Colleges (Liberal Arts)
❖ undergraduate colleges with at least 50 percent of their degrees in liberal arts—5.5%

Baccalaureate Colleges (General)
❖ undergraduate colleges with fewer than 50 percent of their degrees in liberal arts—8.0%

Baccalaureate/Associate's Colleges
❖ undergraduate colleges with a majority of their degrees below the baccalaureate level—1.3%

Associate's Colleges
❖ offer degrees and certificate programs, but no baccalaureate degrees—42.5%

Specialized Institutions
❖ offer degrees from bachelor's to doctoral, with at least half in a single area (e.g., medical schools, seminaries, law schools, business and professional schools)—19.2%

Tribal Colleges
❖ tribally controlled and located on reservations—0.7%

Adapted from Basinger, 2000

FIGURE 4.1
Carnegie Foundation's Reclassification of 3,856 Colleges and Universities

Given these and many other internal and external factors, how does a department position itself to survive and thrive in higher education? To put it simply, the field of health, kinesiology, and leisure studies (HKLS) must increase its centrality to the university community. Think of centrality as you would a sociogram. A sociogram is constructed (often in school classrooms) by asking a group of individuals to indicate other individuals in the group whom they like and with whom they want to interact (e.g., play, work). An oval represents each individual, with lines extending toward and out from these ovals, depending on the individual's selections. If two people select each other, then the line connecting their ovals has arrows on both ends. Suppose a sociogram were constructed for the departments in your university, with regard to their importance (figure 4.2). How many departments would list HKLS as important to their own functioning and success? Would HKLS appear as in figure 4.2, where lines extend away from it to other units, but none are pointed back toward it?

FIGURE 4.2.
Sample Sociogram
of Academic
Departments

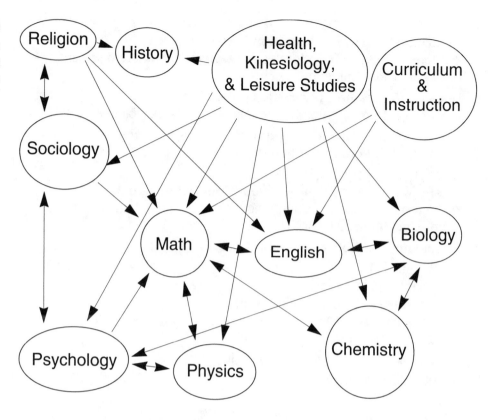

Becoming Central to Your University

Suppose figure 4.2 were based on interdisciplinary research efforts or on overall contributions to the university's mission—how would HKLS fare?

Mission. Develop a unique mission that is important to your college and university (Scanlon, 1998). This mission should explain why the department's activities are important, and to whom they are important. Every faculty member should know this mission. For example, the mission of kinesiology is the study of physical activity. This mission can be adapted in unique ways that best fit your institutional culture. In general, though, we must be faculty who study, teach, and promote physical activity, not faculty who use physical activity as a medium through which to test theories from other fields (e.g., psychology, sociology). That is what separates an exercise physiologist from a physiologist or a sport psychologist from a psychologist. If the university community cannot understand why an exercise physiologist is different from a physiologist, then no reason exists to house them in separate academic units. If exercise physiologists are subsumed by physiology departments, they may or may not be replaced with exercise physiologists when they retire or otherwise vacate their positions, depending on the interests and needs of the physiology departments.

Critical Mass of Faculty. As Scanlon (1998) put it, "several physiologists and a small smattering of faculty in a few other areas 'do not a kinesiology department make'" (pp. 130-131). The results of that strategy have clearly been found wanting. A balance of faculty across academic content areas creates better ties to other areas in the university and increases the department's centrality. Fragmenting into small and ineffective units is political suicide on most campuses[2]. Thus, having faculty in sport and exercise psychology, health, sport sociology, physical education, biomechanics, leisure studies, sport management, athletic training, motor behavior, health promotion and exercise, and other areas provides a broader mission, more faculty connections, more opportunities for cross- and inter-disciplinary research, and greater appreciation for the field of HKLS. However, if you want to be eliminated or absorbed into another academic unit, then:

1. Elect and reelect a weak chair.
2. Lose your most productive colleagues to other institutions.
3. Eschew undergraduate education and majors.
4. Forego participation in campus governance.
5. Glory in bitter ideological and personal vendettas.
6. When all else fails, war against your dean.

From Abler (1992)

Wilmore (1998) reported the results of a survey of the Fellows in the American Academy of Kinesiology and Physical Education concerning those characteristics that determine a department's success or failure:

Characteristics or attributes of a department and/or its faculty that are important for survival and academic excellence in today's academic and economic environment

Characteristics for Survival

Internal to the Department

1. Departmental administration
   - Publicize and defend program
   - Get faculty to pull together
2. Faculty
   - Respect and support colleagues in other departmental subdisciplines
   - Demonstrate a high level of scholarship
   - Be productive (i.e., publish in "good" journals and obtain external funding for research)
   - Be committed to teaching excellence (at undergraduate and graduate levels)
   - Value the disciplinary and professional aspects of the field
   - Maintain a balance between research and teaching
3. Students
   - Recruit and graduate high-quality (academically strong) students
   - Maintain high enrollments
4. Programs
   - Develop a clear program mission statement and strategic plan for achieving this mission (mission should be consistent with the objectives of the university)
   - Ensure that curriculum is unique within the university, up-to-date, and rigorous
   - Offer courses that are attractive and lead to a marketable degree

- Provide unique services and courses to others (i.e., a course that meets university general education requirements or also services students in another major)
- Offer a strong graduate program with high academic standards that is led by faculty with national reputations in the subdisciplines
- Strive to obtain and offer more postdoctoral opportunities

External to the Department

1. Administration: Department administrator's roles within the university
   - Promote and publicize the department's programs and faculty on campus
   - Locate and cultivate higher-level administrators who know about and support the department
   - Maintain visibility in seeking additional resources for the department
   - Have the courage to defend the department's programs to top administrators
2. Faculty: Faculty members' roles within the university
   - Interact with faculty in other disciplines on programmatic issues and courses
   - Be politically active on campus (i.e., serve on university-wide committees, review boards, and faculty governance groups)
   - Become involved with cross-campus faculty-development opportunities, teaching workshops, and interdisciplinary programs
3. Programs
   - Evaluate programs continually to assure that they are central to the mission of the university
   - Be willing to change with the times
   - Maintain quality and rigor of programs so that they are respected both on campus and by professional colleagues, nationally and internationally

External to the University

1. Administration and faculty
   - Become visible and involved within the community by providing services valuable to citizens and offering active outreach programs
   - Develop strong, active, and interested alumni by keeping in touch with students graduating from the department's undergraduate and graduate programs
   - Encourage faculty to become involved and visible in the profession—locally, nationally, and internationally

Characteristics or attributes of a department and/or its faculty that might contribute to its demise in today's academic and economic environment

Characteristics Contributing to Demise

1. Department
   - Small faculty or too few tenured faculty
   - Low or declining enrollments
   - Poor-quality students
   - Low academic standards
   - Weak graduate program
   - Weak undergraduate program
   - Isolation from other academic units, the university as a whole, and the community
   - Lack of balance within the department (focus on only one or two areas)
   - Dissociated curriculum
   - Resistance to changing curriculum despite a changing market
   - Inappropriate department location
   - Insufficient budget and poor budget management
2. Leadership
   - Poor leadership (ineffective representation of department to higher administration)
   - Lack of vision for the future
   - Minimal campus visibility for the department
   - Lack of communication regarding department value to campus
   - Lack of . . . forward-thinking mission
3. University or college view of department
   - Not seen as central to the mission of the university (lacking centrality)
   - Not liked by administration
   - Equated with athletics
   - Not seen as contributing to the general education requirements for the university
4. Faculty
   - Inadequate scholarship
   - Limited external funding
   - Internal fighting, disunity, and lack of full support of all departmental programs
   - Lack of entrepreneurship
   - Faculty trained in other fields
   - Insecurity
   - Lack of faculty visibility on campus and at national and international levels
5. External factors
   - No jobs for students
   - Decreased support for physical education in public schools

From Wilmore (1998, pp. 105-107)

Of course not all of these characteristics will apply to every situation. Deans will vary in what they expect from departments and in the way they represent their colleges/schools within the university community. How a college of liberal arts and sciences positions itself will differ from how a professional college positions itself. In addition, colleges/schools/departments will vary considerably according to the type of institution in which they reside. Some of the values that are important in research universities will differ from those that are important in regional or liberal arts institutions. Institutions of the same type will also differ from each other. However, many of the characteristics reported by Wilmore will apply across different types of institutions.

How Chairs Can Help Their Units Survive

As has been pointed out by past surveys and expert opinion, leadership is an essential factor if HKLS units are to survive and thrive in higher education. Of course for good leadership to matter, the critical items discussed previously are essential—strong faculty, good students, research productivity, excellence in teaching, and professional service and outreach. However, even with all these factors present, departments can flounder under poor leadership. An essential part of good leadership is the leader's visibility on campus as she/he promotes the department: "Chairs who identify themselves primarily as leaders find great satisfaction in leading capable, competitive teams of faculty, and strive to promote their departments as outstanding and respected entities on campus" (Gmelch & Miskin, 1995, p. 10). In fact, Gmelch and Miskin provided a David-Letterman-style "top ten list" (one hopes in jest) of reasons why professors become chairs:

10. Because you don't want someone else to do it even if you don't.
9. Because you are burned out teaching the same thing over and over again for 20 years and writing articles [that] two people in the whole country read.
8. For the money.
7. For the petty power, having in middle age experienced a precipitous decline...and needing an alternative thrill.
6. Because you lack imagination and can't think of anything better and more original to do.
5. Because you have imagination and fantasize about all the things you will do...to your peers that they did to you while they were chair.
4. Because some dean has made you an offer you can't refuse.
3. Because your peers elect you [in order] to slow down your rate-busting activity by loading you up with administrative trivia.
2. Because your peers elect you, thinking you are useless at research and teaching....this way, you can at least fill [out] administrative reports.
1. Because you temporarily became insane, forgetting why you came into academics in the first place, momentarily...mistaking your little college or university for General Motors or Microsoft, thinking you will climb the ladder."

From Gmelch & Miskin (1995, p. 3)

Administrators of academic units can take several actions to promote their unit and its value to the university community. To some extent, departmental administrators serve as double agents: they must promote and represent the faculty and staff to the dean and, at the same time, represent the dean and the higher administration to the faculty and staff. Walking this line requires a skilled acrobat (administrator) who can gain the trust and support of both sides. First and foremost, the faculty and the dean must have confidence in the honesty and integrity of the chair. Unless the double agent performs well, the significance, centrality, and even the existence of the department is "at risk." Successful chairs do four things well: faculty development, management, leadership, and scholarship (Gmelch & Miskin, 1995).

Following are some additional strategies that I have gleaned from observing chairs who were effective within their academic communities:

- *Keep the dean and the faculty informed*—Neither the dean nor faculty members like academic or personal surprises. Give the dean or faculty members a "heads up" if you think something might be coming their way: at least they will have some planning time. Also, keep the dean and faculty posted on good things that are happening in your unit through regular memos and e-mails.
- *Balance competition with cooperation*—Chairs within a college need to compete for resources, but this can be done with a cooperative spirit—consider what is best for everyone. There are only so many resources, and your unit cannot have all of them. Be fair and objective—this will increase the respect that other units have for you and your department.
- *Form an effective working group in your college*—Chairs in the same college can develop respect and regard for each other by holding a social event (e.g., a breakfast) once per month. This can result in the formation of professional friendships and trust that lead to cooperative planning, particularly with regard to the use of resources.
- *Keep up your scholarship*— The average tenure of a chair is six years: Gmelch and Miskin (1995) use the phrase "as the chair swivels" to describe this fact. Sixty-five percent of chairs return to the faculty (p. 129). Nobody needs a faculty member who has lost his or her scholarly skills while serving as chair: this benefits neither the department, the university, nor the academic field.
- *Administer by walking around*—This is not advice on how to help your department survive in the university; it is my personal advice to you as a chair. Get a cup of coffee first thing every morning and walk around in your department—stop and talk to the faculty, staff, and students you meet. It's amazing how much you will learn and how sensitive you will become to developing issues.

I would also like to share one moment from my history as a chair that turned out well. It occurred when I first came to chair the Department of Health and Human Performance at Iowa State University in 1998. I had previously been a chair at both Louisiana State University and Arizona State University (some wags would say because I can't get it right). Soon after arriving, I found myself in a meeting of department chairs (who also carry the title of "department executive officer," or DEO, at Iowa State) and the dean of our college. DEOs are organized into the DEO Council, which elects a DEO Cabinet as the governing body. This group serves as advisor to the provost and plans DEO training on campus. Each college elects one DEO to the Cabinet, and there are an additional four at-large DEOs elected. When the dean asked for volunteers, I agreed to serve because I thought it would be a good way to get to know other DEOs on campus. In my second year in the DEO Cabinet, I was elected Chair of the Cabinet. As a result, I had the opportunity to do a number of things, including:

- planning the university-wide new-DEO training in cooperation with the Provost's Office;
- organizing and participating in a university-wide program (and developing a manual) to prepare DEOs to aggressively address issues of sexual and racial harassment that might occur in their departments;
- serving on a search committee for the Vice Provost for Research and Graduate Studies, who turned out to be the person I nominated and who has an appointment in my department; and
- serving on the search committee for the new university president.

Certainly a case for good fortune can be made here—a number of significant events occurred while I was a part of the DEO Cabinet. However, I would never have had those opportunities had I not volunteered to be in the Cabinet when the dean asked. Participating in these events has helped me establish a leadership role on campus and increase the visibility of my department.

Summary

Previously, I have pointed out that *prominence within the academic field is nice, but prominence within the university community is essential* (Thomas, 1998). Singer (1998) noted that kinesiology has moved from a peripheral to a central role in the university because of interest in exercise, health, and sports, and the importance of movement to daily life. It's great if everyone (nationally and internationally) knows about your department's faculty, research, and students. However, long-term departmental health is influenced more by what your local departments, deans, and university administrators know about your role in these activities. To survive, we need to know the rules of the centrality "game." Krahenbuhl (1998) provided the rules for the internal health of a department and discipline (as least as he sees them, as dean of a large college of arts and sciences):

- Expect change and exploit it
- Expect universities to value and reward responsiveness to institutional needs
- Prepare future faculty with a sense of stewardship for their field and institutions
- Expect to be undervalued and take steps to build your indispensability to your campus, region, and nation. (pp. 114-115)

Notes

1. Because of recent changes in some of the traditionally strong programs, it is difficult to make judgments about them. For example, Pennsylvania State University has eliminated its stand-alone college in our field, but the individual Department of Kinesiology still appears strong. Another example is the renowned Department of Kinesiology at the University of Illinois at Urbana-Champaign; they have recently lost several senior faculty to retirement or to other institutions, and it is unclear how that will influence their future.

2. I'm not suggesting that HKLS has to be one academic unit. Often, these are separate academic units that have the size and scope to stand alone. What I am suggesting is that units in kinesiology that fragment into subsets (e.g., exercise science, sport and leisure, physical education) are generally making an error because of their small size.

About the Author

Jerry R. Thomas is a professor in, and Chair of, the Department of Health and Human Performance at Iowa State University. He has previously served as both a chair and a dean at Arizona State University, and as a chair at Louisiana State University.

References

Abler, R. (1992). Six steps to oblivion. *Association of American Geographers Newsletter*. Washington, DC.

Almanac. (1999). *Chronicle of Higher Education, 46*(1), 7-29.

Basinger, J. (2000, August 11). A new way of classifying colleges elates some and perturbs others. *Chronicle of Higher Education, 66*(49), A31, A34-A42.

Gmelch, W. H., & Miskin, V. D. (1995). *Chairing the academic department*. Thousand Oaks, CA: Sage.

Krahenbuhl, G. S. (1998). Higher education in the 21st century: The role of kinesiology and physical education. *Quest, 50*, 108-115.

Scanlon, T. K. (1998). Thriving versus surviving. *Quest, 50*, 126-133.

Singer, R. N. (1998). Gaining identity and respect for a department. *Quest, 50*, 149-158.

Thomas, J. R. (1998). Arizona State University: Prominence within the university is essential; Prominence within the academic field is nice. *Quest, 50*, 159-165.

Wilmore, J. H. (1998). Building strong academic programs for our future. *Quest, 50*, 103-107.

SECTION II

Realities and Theories of Managing and Leading

5 Applying Theories of Management

Hally B. W. Poindexter, *Professor Emeritus, Rice University*

Understand that most situations are not truly crises. So, take time to analyze and prioritize before responding.

James E. Bryant

For those of us who began our administrative and management experiences in health, kinesiology, and leisure studies (HKLS) prior to the 1990s, our degrees of success were largely dependent on our individual styles, skills, and intuitions. When we gathered to discuss administrative effectiveness, the conversations began with a clear understanding of line-and-staff organizational charts and a reaffirmation of administrative bureaucracy. For a department chair, there was a direct line of responsibility to the dean, provost, selected vice presidents, and the university president. The dean was the interface between the chair and the higher administrative echelon. Deans were viewed as administrators, while chairs were managers. "Manage" was the verb that indicated what we did with facilities, funds, and personnel issues. Each of us had our own personal philosophies that included the way we dealt with people and the outcome we wanted for our administrative unit. These philosophies constituted a stylistic continuum that served as a model of measurement, a yardstick, for every administrator. A controlling, bureaucratic style was reflected at one end of the continuum, and a casual, laissez-faire attitude at the other end, with many variations in between. There was the dictatorial, arbitrary, and unyielding administrator, and the "laid back" manager who let things flow until it was suggested that there might be a problem requiring intervention. Both administrators may have had leadership and management success, and both may have had failures and critics. In defense of both, they were simply following the pattern of the day; their styles were founded on educational and psychological theories, principles, and management

45

techniques that were accepted at the time. To understand how management and administration came into education and how they have changed over the years, one must look at the history of management in American business.

"Management" became a watchword following the Industrial Revolution, when men left their hand-crafted tools and home shops for factories and industrial manufacturing operations. Laborers were brought together under one roof in the factories, and manufacturing processes were watched over by supervisors. It was soon observed that expanded mechanization and complexity of operations were accompanied by much waste and inefficiency. In an effort to improve profits and minimize material waste, time-motion studies became a feature of shop management. Over time, these studies taught the overseers (management) to take into account the limits of human physical and mental capacities and the importance of a good physical environment (e.g., good lighting, heating, and ventilation). It was an impartial and impersonal system that did not adjust its procedures or its outcomes to individual differences and favoritism. There were clear lines of control and responsibility in this model; information flowed upward and decisions flowed downward. Clearly, this pattern could be viewed in many universities and departments of health, physical education, and recreation as late as the 1960s.

As America entered the 20th century, education, operating independently of business, felt little alignment with the corporate focus on profit; its core concern was the educational development of individuals. Educational leaders determined that the developing "business model" of management had little place in education. It remained for educators to develop their own administrative mechanisms and styles in order to enhance learning. Since educational institutions enjoyed constitutional protection from governmental management, they proudly maintained political, academic, and territorial independence, and their administrative styles reflected these differences.

By the late 20th century, however, numerous events had motivated educators to examine the corporate world for management ideas. The corporate world's newfound concern for the human element provided evidence that factors other than time-motion studies and improved production lines should be considered in the quest for increased profits. Given the success and failure of various management techniques and ideas, a concept of "management theory" took root. Theories are little more than speculation, but they are based on observations, pragmatic evidence, principles both proven and suggested, and a myriad of ideas both borrowed and original. Although theories are generally well thought out, they may also be little more than well-educated and designed guesses about how management should work. The most interesting developments of early management theory in education were the growing concern for the human element and the notion of management as a "science." This was of particular interest to department chairs in HKLS, who were aware of the importance of the human element in education long before their colleagues in other fields. Administrators in these fields were often called upon by higher administrative authorities to explain ways of addressing human needs in the curricula of higher education.

Harwood F. Merrill's *Classics in Management* (1960) cited works from authors who contributed "classic" works in management theory and model development. Tracing these scholarly treatises, there appears to be a straight-line progression in—and a cohesive picture of—management philosophy from the 1800s well into the 20th century. This progressive pathway began with Babbage's analytical approach to factory methods and costs as exemplified in his essay on the division of labor. Metcalfe brought the word "science" into the world of management in 1885, stating that "the administration of arsenals and other workshops is on great measure an art and depends upon the application to a great variety of cases of certain principles, which taken together make up what may be called the science of administration" (Merrill, p. 13). Taylor, Gantt, and Brandeis coined the term "scientific management" in 1910, and Taylor stated that management would become an organized body of knowledge. In 1920, Robert Owen noted that a change in management philosophy was evident. Following Gantt—who addressed the need for winning the cooperation of workers and insisted that good management meant leading rather than driving—Owen introduced the concept of the human element in management. Since that time, management philosophy, theories, and models have moved steadily toward recognizing the importance of the human factor. So integral is this human factor in today's world that a new market for labor and procurement services has spawned. This 21st-century growth industry, "Human Capital Management," is the business of hiring and handling employees across major areas of business, education, and government.

As educational administrators became aware that business models were becoming more humane and education was becoming more akin to business, programs in health, physical education, recreation, dance, and athletics were among the first to embrace new management theories and styles. The transition was slow, as seen in the fourth edition of Williams and Brownell's (1951) best-selling administrative textbook, *The Administration of Health and Physical Education*. This text identified four areas of administrative concern in the fields, and the percentage of material that the authors devoted to each topic is indicative of the administrative value placed on each area: leadership, 19 percent; program, 43 percent; physical facilities, 24 percent; community, state, and legal issues, 14 percent. Fiduciary affairs and personnel development are notable only for their absence. However, it was clear that educators needed to be concerned with both materialistic and humanistic products. Athletics had already moved into the realm of business, and all of education was in need of accountability and evaluation. There was evidence, and a few educators who were believers, that the concept of scientific management might be worthy of pursuit.

Serious focus on the human element in management was presented in Douglas McGregor's 1960 book, *The Human Side of Enterprise*, which postulated two major theories. "Theory X" holds that the average human has an inherent dislike for work and will avoid it if possible. Theory X views individuals as oriented toward material rewards and prone to ride on the effort of others when given an opportunity. Acceptance of this theory by many business organizations and some educational leaders implied their belief that workers preferred to be told what to do rather than accept responsibility or manifest ambition. These assumptions led to the "us vs. them" concept of management.

"Theory Y" took the opposite position; it stated that work was a natural behavior and that the average person finds it to be a source of satisfaction. Acceptance of this theory led to the concept that external control and threat of punishment are not the best ways to elicit effort toward an organization's goals. Rather, worker commitment to objectives is a function of rewards associated with achievement and self-actualization. Theory Y held that the individual's capacity for imagination and ingenuity was the solution to organizational problems and that these intellectual potentials should be sought and expanded.

In 1981, William Ouchi proposed "Theory Z," based on the Japanese management style. He suggested that business and education should seek participatory management from employees who are committed to their work due to shared values. Some attribute the slow acceptance of Theory Z to the fact that it was predicated on high levels of trust, long-term job security, and holistic career planning; others suggest that corporate and educational administrators were not ready to share decision-making. Although educational administrators and program organizers in the U.S. were slow to respond to this communal form of management, there were some department chairs in HKLS who were particularly adept at listening to their colleagues, faculty members, and students. Daily interactions with undergraduate and graduate students, along with information gleaned from the playing fields, gymnasiums, and classrooms, all served to challenge the educational goals, methodologies, and leadership styles of these administrators. It was this true participatory management with students and faculty that allowed meaningful changes to occur in our fields.

Reflecting on the last 50 years, there is evidence in both administrative theory and practice that effective management behavior has moved from the authoritarian toward the humane. This was a comfortable shift for HKLS administrators, for ours is a naturally humane field. Our business is the individual, the mind and body, and we have long been sensitive to human needs. This paradigm shift was supported by Deborah Ancona (1999), who characterized the classic model of formal organization prevalent in the 1950s and '60s as overly bureaucratic. The five identifying features of that model are:

1. Clearly defined and specialized individual positions (specific job descriptions spelled out the requirements and performance expectations for each individual)
2. A formal hierarchy of authority and power
3. Formal rules and standards that governed operating procedures (following these standard operating procedures, or "SOPs," was an imperative of the old model)
4. Clear boundaries of operational domain and power for each department
5. Standardized training, requirements, career paths, and reward systems based on development of defined expertise (career advancement was stable and predictable for those dutifully fulfilling the requirements).

Organizational theorists, many of whom predicted the shift to a "knowledge-based society," provide an academic perspective on the new era in management. Many educational institutions are responding to organizational changes and are focusing on the corporate world for effective new practices. The new model of management can be understood by examining five interacting features:

1. The need for interdependence of individuals, units, and subunits within the organization and with supporting external groups and environments. This tenet is in obvious contrast to the management theory of old, which emphasized clear lines of individual authority and responsibility for managerial autonomy and for protecting the core activities from external intervention.

2. Minimized hierarchical management. That is, a leaner and more effective management that eliminates layers of middle management and seeks empowerment of the operating levels of the organization (some features of Theory Z). In education, it may mean pushing decision-making to the gymnasium, playing fields, and classroom, and decisions about research interests and community-service functions to the departmental or divisional levels.

3. Flexibility that permits the organization to meet the needs of all stakeholders. (In higher education, a stakeholder is each and every person involved in the organization—from the student, parent, university president, trustees, staff, faculty, and community members.) This flexibility in universal public education is allowing communities to consider the values of home schooling programs, charter schools, community colleges, liberal arts institutions, as well as technical institutions.

4. Diversity. The new management model accommodates people with different perspectives and approaches, varied career paths, varying incentive systems, altered work schedules, and widely differing constituencies and stakeholders. Diversity encourages innovation and creativity in approaching the learning and delivery systems and never rules out the potential benefits in new technology, "outsourcing," contract workers, "tele-working," and distance learning.

5. Global. The new theory requires consideration of all of the world. Companies that had operated internationally through sales or products exchange are now actively involved in manufacturing, development, and all aspects of business in many countries. International trade agreements encourage and support international trade and cultural development. It will be the graduates of our institutions that lead our industries across the boundaries of many countries. It is imperative that students be globally prepared by understanding diversity of values, language, culture, and educational goals.

Adapted from Ancona (1999, pp. C8-C12)

Introduction of the new model is proving very difficult for some organizations, and the shift is stressful on employees. The "new" has its problems, and many institutions will continue with the old model for its resilience and employee security. Others will combine old features and new, and for a very few, there will be a major transformation to the new paradigm.

How does an individual prepare for a successful management career as a department chair, a dean, or a divisional vice president in the "new order?" How does an incumbent administrator stay apprised of events and manage in the most effective ways? Does one identify a single model, turn to a specific theory, or go "by the seat of the pants?" Wolcott (2000) wrote of the "cut-and-thrust" world of management described in the plethora of recent books on the subject and directed the reader to new management books that call upon the styles of persons such as Abraham Lincoln, William Shakespeare, and Attila the Hun. He also directed the reader's eyes to the management section of the bookstore, which harbors titles such as *Patton on Leadership: Strategic Lessons for Corporate Warfare*; *Moses on Management*; *What Would Machiavelli Do?*; *Star Trek, the Next Generation: Make It So*; and *The 30 Management Principles of the U.S. Marines*. These writings proclaim effective management and leadership practices for success in the new order.

Filled with faith and confidence, and with my own experiences of walking the bumps and curves of administrative roads as I followed the rainbow over the horizon, I suggest my own plan for management success. Drucker (1973) wrote that the primary dimensions of management were economic performance, making workers productive, and managing social responsibilities and social impact (p. 39). He also stated that the specific work of management is *managing managers*. Transferring Drucker's intent to HKLS, my model is based on the belief that the roles of the college or divisional dean (manager #1) and the department chair (manager #2) are to enhance teaching and scholarly output and promote meaningful departmental, university, community, and professional service. Manager #1 is primarily responsible for finding ways to fund and support the efforts set forth by the team of manager #2. Manager #2 must be in close contact with all of the players involved in the teaching, research, and service endeavors (e.g., faculty, staff, and students). Each administrator must use his or her knowledge and abilities to assure that resources are available for the enhancement of each staff and faculty member's potential contribution to the effectiveness of the unit. I propose a two-phase program that is founded on our knowledge of management theories and paradigms and on our personal environment. In our own "scientific" way, we can develop our own model.

Phase 1. Develop a mission statement for your unit. This must be a cooperative venture that is developed by manager #2's team and approved by manager #1. Begin by assessing what it is that you and your unit can do to fulfill the mission of the institution. This requires a full understanding of that mission and the role of your unit. What are the purposes of the programs in your unit (e.g., basic instruction program, wellness program, professional program, recreational programs)? What about teaching, scholarship, and service? Your answers to these questions should be formed into a "centrality statement" that places the activities of the department at the core of university goals.

Phase 2. The next phase has three "action item" steps bound together by two invasive threads. The threads are labeled "People" (human concerns) and "Things" (all other concerns, such as facilities, funding, etc.). Although curriculum design, money, equipment, and facilities are integral to our programs, it is my contention that if a manager is successful in managing faculty (or other managers), then the "things" will fall into place.

- Step 1—Analyze the responsibilities and performance expectations of the unit manager (e.g., chair, dean) that are necessary to fulfill the teaching mission.
- Step 2—Analyze the responsibilities and performance expectations of the unit manager that are necessary to fulfill the research and scholarly productivity expectations.
- Step 3—Analyze the responsibilities and expectations of the administrator that are necessary to fulfill the service expectations of the department, division, university, community, and professional organizations.

Managers who complete phases 1 and 2 will find an endless list of expectations and obligations unique to their position and setting, from curriculum preparation, to supervision of facility remodeling, to personal scholarly investigations, and so on (my personal list is available on request). Among these responsibilities will be interactions with staff, students, faculty, other administrators, community members, and professionals all across the world.

One way to get a clear picture of what you are currently doing with your time is to generate a record of your actions. All chairs and deans should keep a record of their activities. To begin with, record your daily activities for one "typical" week during each semester. Once a complete week is recorded, examine and evaluate your accomplishments and the efficiency of your time expenditure. Evaluate the effectiveness of your work on personnel issues, curriculum development, facility management, and personnel-improvement programs. Lastly, determine whether you scheduled time to work on visionary thoughts and creative actions.

At the end of a designated time period (e.g., each month or each semester), reflect on your personal management history. What were your successes and misjudgments (*not* failures)? What has been accepted and rejected by the stakeholders (the university administration and faculty)? How has the faculty rated administrative performance in the past? As a personal summation of this evaluation, write about how you have benefited and what you have learned from the process. It will serve as your personal contribution to the field, entitled "wisdom from immersion in the pool of management." My own confessions, lessons, and wisdom gained from administrative experience are summarized below.

Premise:

Sound educational leadership (often referred to as "management" or "administration") is concerned primarily with people. Although technology, facilities, and equipment are of daily concern to the administrator, all issues, solutions, and problems are related to the interactions and adaptive behaviors of people. Good management and leadership in education are directly related to one's ability to work effectively with people.

Self-evident truths:

1. Change is inevitable but may not always be symbolic of progress.
2. To benefit from or respond to changing conditions, people must exhibit adaptive behavior.

3. Experience is relative, personal, and inevitable. We all experience, but do we learn from these experiences? The concept of experience must be carefully analyzed if one is to be certain that 20 years of experience is not really one year of experience repeated 20 times.

4. The turtle on top of the fence post (the administrator) didn't get there by himself, and he won't remain there by his will alone.

Guiding concepts from administrative research:

1. Employees must share values and responsibilities if they are to buy into the program.

2. Participatory management inspires communal decision-making.

3. An empowered work force is characterized by high levels of trust and position security.

4. Successful leaders do not simply provide solutions; leaders must shift the locus of responsibility for problem-solving to the people in the organization. Therefore, position yourself so that these people can see the entire operation. You must be the strategist and the coach who sees the entire court and watches as the plays develop.

5. Educational leaders profit from the study of administrative business models.

Conventional wisdom derived from adages:

1. *Do unto others as you would have them do unto you.* A sincere interest in and concern for people seems imperative in a profession that has the health and well-being of humans at its very core.

2. *Every person has something to offer.* All you need do is simply stop, listen, and share. A truly original idea is rare; we borrow ideas and make creative decisions based on information we glean from others. Everyone you meet and work with can teach you something about dealing with people and issues.

3. *Never ask anyone to do anything that you wouldn't do yourself.* The implication here is not physical effort, but rather your ethics, integrity, and personal demeanor.

4. *You can gather more bees (or grumpy bears) with honey than with vinegar.* Pleasant demeanor, civility, and collegiality are basic requirements for leaders.

5. *Perception is one's view of reality.* People base their beliefs on how they see the world and specific situations. Their perception can be changed only by broadening it through learning or experience. Limited perception results in biases, tunnel vision, and an inability to accept adaptive behaviors.

6. *We grow together or we grow apart.* This valuable statement can apply to individual cooperative endeavors as well as to the development of an entire academic unit. Goals and ideas must be shared if people are to grow together.

7. *What goes around, comes around.* The way you deal with people—your sincerity, integrity, and methods—will be returned to you in time.

8. *Vive la différence (Long live the difference).* Respect diversity of background, creed, race, and thought. We each have unique value; we can be intellectual, creative, cooperative, catalytic, or worker-bee individuals.

9. *To err is human, to forgive, divine.* Administrators quickly learn that action often results in errors, and that inaction results in nothing (i.e., no progress). The encouragement of adaptive behavior and effort will result in errors, but errors can be corrected, and forgiveness must follow.

10. *Respect is not a gift—it is earned.* A leader earns respect through consistent manifestation of honesty, integrity, effort, and concern for colleagues.

11. *"You have my word."* There should be no stronger bond in a personal or professional relationship than complete assurance that you will do what you say you will do!

12. *A desk is a dangerous place from which to view the world.* John le Carre's quote hangs over the desk of IBM CEO Louis Gerstner, Jr. A leader must get out and about learning, understanding, explaining, and interpreting the program, its mission, and the global purpose of educational initiatives.

13. *Equality means everyone.* Considering the advantages of diversity, each person should be treated with an even hand.

14. *If you elect to be a leader, you must ride to the front of the herd!* Administrators must enter the fray of daily events and avoid issuing edicts from afar. If you want to change the course of a wandering (or stampeding!) herd, you must get on a horse and work your way through it to the point position, and then turn the herd in the desired direction.

15. *Work dignifies you: reciprocate!*

16. *Stop and smell the roses.* Encourage your colleagues to join you in a trust-developing experience.

As a final admonition, learn leadership behaviors from your interactions with family, peers, colleagues, supervisors, and all persons whom you encounter in work, play, and religious endeavors. As implied previously, the most important lessons you can learn are those about working with people—how they like to be treated, what you can expect of them, and how they will respond to your behaviors.

Leadership behaviors supported by conventional wisdom:

1. Seek a variety of innovative leadership opportunities. Experience all venues.

2. Seek mentors who can impart lessons of patience, ethical behavior, integrity, fairness, and civility.

3. Learn the art of persuasion. It is far more lasting and effective than dictatorial leadership, which orders and directs and builds barriers to those with different opinions. Persuasion is an educational endeavor that requires research, fact determination, and the ability to convey this information in a way related to the issues at hand. When successful, persuasion wins not only the vote but the commitment and confidence of the one persuaded.

4. Develop your special intellectual potential. There are many forms of intelligence and manifestations of intelligent behavior. Learn and develop your strong suits while learning to value people with different potentials.

5. Develop and use wit and humor effectively.

6. Treat people with dignity and trust.
7. Seek an understanding of new initiatives and creative agendas. This may be done through membership on committees or task forces that have the potential for major impact within the university. Assuming the leadership role of a major accreditation committee or a university committee on strategic planning may have a positive outcome for you and your department.
8. Avail yourself of opportunities to learn leadership styles and processes through formal training programs. One is never too old or too secure in leadership skills to benefit from such training.
9. Have fun and enjoy people. A strong leader encourages fun and pleasurable interaction among employees and constituencies.

Today's successful managers motivate people to fulfill their potential while contributing to the common goals of the organization. Managing is an art, a science, and a profession. We study it, practice it, and analyze it. It is a vibrant and changing field, and many of us in education will continue to explore management theories and behaviors in the hopes of finding guidelines for productive and responsible leadership. Accept the challenge and enjoy the chase!

About the Author

Hally B. W. Poindexter, Professor Emeritus, Rice University, has held administrative positions in three universities in the areas of health, kinesiology, and student affairs. Prior to retirement, she served for 17 years as Chair of the Department of Human Performance and Health Sciences at Rice University.

References

Ancona, D. (1999). *Managing for the future*. Cincinnati, OH: South-Western College Publishing.

Drucker, P. F. (1973). *Management: Tasks, responsibilities, practices*. New York: Harper and Row.

McGregor, D. (1960). *The human side of enterprise*. New York: McGraw Hill.

Merrill, H. F. (Ed.). (1960). *Classics in management*. New York: American Management Association.

Ouchi, W. G. (1981). *Theory Z: How American business can meet the Japanese challenge*. Reading, MA: Addison Wesley.

Williams, J. F., & Brownell, C. (1951). *The administration of health and physical education* (4th ed.). Philadelphia: W. B. Saunders.

Wolcott, J. (2000, June). How to succeed in business without really breathing. *Vanity Fair (no. 478)*, 62-72.

6 Socialization within an Academic Unit: Working Toward a Common Ground

Judith A. Bischoff, *Professor and Chair, Department of Kinesiology and Physical Education, Northern Illinois University*

When you face the sand storms, thunderstorms, and hailstorms and venting storms remain calm.

⊶ Judith A. Bischoff

Higher education contains a culture different from that of other institutions and corporations. The academic world supports values, mores, beliefs, and attitudes that, while similar to those supported outside academia, are peculiar to its own unique structure. Each individual institution of higher education is also unique within the academic world, and within each such institution is a variety of subcultures, the department being one.

While there is an expectation that individual departments will develop policies, procedures, missions, goals, and strategic plans that are congruent with the institution's own, there is also an acknowledgement that these units often make their own unique contributions to academia. Subcultures are supported by institutions as long as their differences fall within a range deemed acceptable by these institutions.

Tierney (1989, 1993) and Van Patten (1990) have examined important aspects of academic life by emphasizing various cultural elements. Identification of student subcultures and group associations has been a principal area of such cultural investigation. More recent work has examined academic institutions in a more holistic fashion, treating the institution itself as an organized culture. Cultural research has also focused on the multiple roles adopted by faculty that reflect their own learning experiences—in other words, their socialization.

Socialization is a concept that has concerned social scientists throughout the 20th century and into the present. For some, it is a means of achieving a sense of solidarity through the institutionalization of shared values. For others, socialization is a means of reproducing the mores of the dominant culture at the expense of alternative ones. Some theorists have investigated socialization as a common need across cultures, and others have considered the interaction between the individual psyche and the social organization. Many anthropologists have thought of some forms of socialization as ritualized processes that involve the transmission of culture.

Socialization within higher education should be viewed as a reciprocal process, in that it produces changes in individuals as well as in departments and institutions (Tierney & Rhoads, 1993). The values, beliefs, and attitudes held by faculty reflect their socialization experiences, and these faculty in turn create their department's culture.

Socialization also occurs implicitly and explicitly. For faculty, implicit socialization may occur around the water cooler, in the locker room, on the golf course, over lunch, or at various social gatherings. Implicit socialization is difficult to observe and analyze, for it occurs spontaneously and unobtrusively. Explicit socialization involves clearly delineated cultural structures such as promotion and tenure procedures and expectations, sabbaticals, merit criteria, and perceived or expressed responsibilities for teaching, research, and service.

Although it occurs most clearly when new faculty enter an institution, college, or department, socialization is an ongoing process. Each type of institution (e.g., community college; liberal arts college; comprehensive, doctoral, or research institution) also offers different cultural climates and, hence, different expectations. Regardless, for new faculty, organizational socialization is the process of learning the ropes (Tierney & Rhoads, 1993), being trained, and being taught what is important in any given department, college, and university.

The primary focus of a new faculty member is the department and, in some cases, a subdiscipline within the department. In turn, senior faculty and the department chair play critical roles in the departmental socialization process. Tierney and Rhoads (1993) view the socialization of faculty as a two-stage process: the anticipatory stage and the organizational stage.

Anticipatory Socialization

Anticipatory socialization pertains to how nonmembers take on the attitudes, actions, and values of the group to which they aspire. During graduate school, students learn (either formally or through personal observation) the behaviors they need to exhibit in order to succeed as faculty members. Graduate training is where students begin to acquire the values, norms, attitudes, and beliefs associated with their area of study (which could take the form of a subculture) and with the profession in general. As Anderson and Seashore-Louis have indicated, "As young scholars work with professors, they observe and internalize the norms of behavior for research as well as supporting mechanisms such as peer review and academic freedom" (cited in Tierney & Rhoads, 1993, p. 24).

Graduate training serves as a significant force in socializing students into the roles and expectations associated with becoming part of academia. Initially, how one interacts with students and colleagues, the lifestyle one leads, the conferences one attends, and the journals and books that one reads are all learned from assigned mentors, senior faculty, peers in graduate school, and personal observation. However, the socializing experiences that new faculty bring from their graduate institutions or previous departments may not necessarily match the culture of their new department. Thus socialization should begin prior to a new faculty member's first day of employment. The department's faculty—especially the senior faculty and, to some degree, the chair—have significant control over the structures that frame the department experience, the department culture, and the department climate. The current faculty have a responsibility to assist new faculty in learning the department ethos.

The organizational stage has two phases: initial entry and role continuance. The first involves interaction during the recruitment and selection process, as well as the early period of learning that occurs when new faculty members enter the department. The role-continuance phase begins after new faculty are situated. The organizational stage is initially framed by activities that occurred during anticipatory socialization and that have helped shape a new faculty member's responses to task demands and professional performance requirements (Tierney & Rhoads, 1993).

Organizational Socialization

When the anticipatory socialization of new faculty is consistent with the new department's culture, they will experience organizational socialization that affirms the qualities they have brought to the department. On the other hand, if their values, beliefs, and norms are seen as inconsistent with the cultural ethos of the department, then the socialization experience will be more transformative. The department will attempt to modify, perhaps significantly, the new faculty members' values and beliefs to match more closely the culture of the department.

Once new faculty members are hired, they may experience unique problems and concerns. As Baldwin has indicated, "The new professor's major concern is competence….This entry period is a time of intense pressure and considerable growth" (cited in Tierney & Rhoads, 1993, p. 35). Graduate-school days are left behind, and new faculty members enter the professoriate as novices attempting to understand the rites of passage needed to become full members of the faculty. New faculty coming from other institutions are also novices to the department attempting to learn their roles. In this process, struggles and conflicts will be evident as all new faculty sort out their past experiences and the expectations of their new department. This early socialization is not just a formalized process; it also requires that complex and varied social norms be learned. For example, new faculty will find themselves asking questions such as: What is the role of new faculty at faculty meetings? Who sits where? What are the social customs at informal faculty gatherings? Who is approachable for assistance with classes? Who are the senior faculty members, and are they approachable? What are the "turf" issues in the department regarding curriculum, laboratory space, use of equipment, and so forth? Should I ask to go to lunch with other faculty members? Where can I park? Do I need a parking sticker? Where is the library, and what is the process for putting materials on reserve? Which office is mine, and will I be sharing with another faculty member? How do I get keys? Will I have a computer? How do I get my e-mail account? Where do I get my mail? How does the phone system work?

Just as new faculty attempt to learn the department culture, so have senior faculty moved through these rites of passage and, in essence, helped shape the department culture. Thus, the senior faculty tend to serve as socializers, usually on an informal basis, for the new faculty. Tierney and Rhoads (1993) presented three roles that senior faculty fill in their capacity as socializers and bearers of the department culture: symbolic leader, trail guide, and oral historian.

As symbolic leaders, senior faculty set standards by example. A full professor who seeks out a junior colleague for honest advice about an article on which he or she is working, or a department chair who solicits input from junior faculty about the nature of the curriculum, are each demonstrating to new faculty that their ideas are important and will be considered.

As trail guides, senior faculty may find that less experienced faculty seek their advice about the cultural mores of the department (e.g., "How often am I expected to be in my office?" "Do I keep the door open or closed when I am there?" "Is there a dress code for teaching class?" "Is it permissible to just walk into other faculty members' offices?"). Some of these questions are asked and answered in informal conversations around the mailbox, in the hallway, or on the way to conferences. These serve as implicit indicators to new faculty of the department's culture. Such questions and conversations may seem trivial, but they form the core of the implicit cultural weavings that bind department faculty members. Senior faculty can create an inclusive culture wherein the new faculty members' interests are heard and honored, or they can create an exclusive environment to emphasize that a hierarchical structure exists.

As oral historians, senior faculty can provide important information (that does not appear in any written materials) about life in the department and about the department's role in the college and university. This knowledge is contained in the myths that pass from one faculty generation to another. Myth here indicates a narrative of events that often have a sacred quality. Myths link the present to the past; therefore, based on their years in academia and their experiences at specific institutions, senior faculty hold the keys to a wealth of institutional myths. This includes departmental myths, which can reveal much about the cultural fabric of the department.

Senior faculty can be instrumental in socializing all new faculty, or they can be more selective in their interactions, leaving new faculty to learn the ropes on their own. The latter approach will force new faculty to rely on: the socialization processes they experienced in graduate school or at another institution; the information in the department faculty handbook (if there is one); or other pieces of written material having little if any relationship to the unwritten rules, and which may or may not fit the department culture. Many senior faculty are comfortable with the values, mores, and attitudes into which they were socialized, and which they helped establish in the department. While this is a valid attitude, new faculty could bring different perspectives that are worthy of consideration. This is especially true if there are large numbers of department retirements or resignations in a short period of time. Once the symbolic leaders, experienced trail guides, and oral historians are gone, both the department and new faculty are left to be shaped by the younger faculty.

However, there should be some common values that last across generations—values that younger faculty have learned from senior faculty and that maintain the department ethos. But as time goes by, departments may feel the need for change that could alter the department culture (e.g., acquiring a doctoral program, dropping a program, focusing on outreach programs, all of which are likely to change a number of factors in the department). The department chair must play a critical role in the socialization of new faculty and in the development of the department's culture. Since not all senior faculty interpret the department culture in the same way, the department chair can serve as a "clearinghouse" for interpretation. If the chair was appointed from among the faculty, then she or he should understand the department climate and be able to provide some continuity to the department culture. If the chair is a recent appointee from outside the department, however, she or he may not understand the faculty well enough to know the implicit factors in the socialization process.

The department chair must also realize that individual departments, though vulnerable to the overall campus climate, can exhibit conditions that are very different from the campus environment. Chairs can influence the department climate through their own managerial actions. Thus chairs need to recognize how their own behavior influences the department climate and how the climate, in turn, facilitates or impedes their ability to manage conflict effectively (Higgerson, 1998). In any department, conflict is inevitable, and the resolution to conflict belongs in the hands of both the faculty and the chair. However, Higgerson indicates that the chair should accept "conflict management" as a goal rather than "conflict resolution": "Conflict management, unlike conflict resolution, acknowledges that human interaction is dynamic and that people do not always think alike. Because conflict results from differences in attitudes, beliefs, and expectations, a conflict-free environment would be one that is so homogeneous that it could not be optimally innovative or productive" (p. 55).

There are several strategies that a chair can use to help new faculty understand the department culture. In doing so, the chair would be attempting to steer potential conflict toward more positive faculty interactions.

- In the interview stage, expectations for new faculty should be clearly defined, preferably by the chair. This is especially important as it relates to promotion, tenure, teaching, research, service, and the curriculum process.
- In their first year, all new faculty should be organized into a group that meets with the chair once a month. This would provide opportunities for clarification and also build a working relationship among new faculty. If there is only one new faculty member, he or she could join the group of faculty who arrived the year before.
- A group of senior faculty members could be identified who would take a new faculty member under their wing, not necessarily in a formal mentorship but rather as an informal association for department cultural orientation. This group might consist of one senior faculty member in the same subject area as the new member, one who may have similar recreation interests, one who is several years from retirement, and one of the same gender or ethnic group. This will also help those in the group get to know one another better; hence, when conflict does arise, the group might tend to have a more positive focus.
- The chair should work with each new faculty member to set yearly goals. These goals should be discussed early in the fall and reviewed at the end of the semester during the progress-toward-tenure meeting. The chair might also consider working with all faculty to set yearly

goals so that he or she has a sense of what all faculty wish to achieve and of how these goals fit into the direction of the department.

- The chair should schedule periodic social events for faculty that facilitate implicit socialization. While it is unlikely that all faculty will attend, it is an important interactive opportunity for those who do.
- The chair should work with senior faculty who may need to be socialized into new roles (e.g., the transition from junior to senior faculty member). Various development options (e.g., computer skills, internet, using technology in the classroom, new programmatic initiatives) may need to be explored to help senior faculty keep up with a changing department culture.

In addition, the chair should be prepared to manage conflict as change occurs, whether between or among junior and senior faculty, between the chair and faculty, or between faculty in difference disciplines or subcultures. Conflict is best managed when it is addressed as soon as it occurs. Academic culture, with its propensity to avoid and deny, often creates faculty who either ignore the issues, hoping that they will disappear, or rush to make a snap judgment. One measure of chairs' effectiveness as leaders is the degree to which they can make sound judgment calls about the importance of an emergent conflict, as well as the timing of their subsequent actions (Sturnick, 1998).

There are many methods that chairs can use in conflict situations. Chairs must create a climate where conflict is perceived as normal, where faculty are encouraged to openly express their views and debate issues in a constructive manner, and where faculty are empowered to solve their own disputes as much as possible (Berryman-Fink, 1998). The sources of conflict among faculty are always present; faculty find themselves arguing over disciplinary turf, curriculum issues, tenure decisions, authorship issues, and the interpretation of academic freedom. Chairs must understand how conflict arises in academia and be familiar with a wide range of conflict-management strategies.

Summary   Integrating new faculty into an existing department culture calls for an understanding of faculty roles and responsibilities at the institution, in the college, and in the department. Socialization and re-socialization are part of that process: new faculty are socialized into the department culture, while senior faculty may need to be re-socialized. The department chair needs to be prepared to work with faculty from different subcultures within the same department. Through some strategic planning, communication, social events, and concerted efforts on the part of faculty members and the chair, a common ground can be established on which to work. Thus when conflict does arise, it can be channeled in a positive direction so that the chair, working with the faculty, can move ahead toward a creative, productive future.

About the Author   Judith A. Bischoff is a professor in, and Chair of, the Department of Kinesiology and Physical Education at Northern Illinois University. She has been with the department for 25 years.

References

Berryman-Fink, C. (1998). Can we agree to disagree? Faculty-faculty conflict. In S. A. Holton (Ed.), *Mending the cracks in the ivory tower: Strategies for conflict management in higher education* (pp. 141-163). Boston: Anker.

Higgerson, M. L. (1998). Chairs as department managers: Working with support staff. In S. A. Holton (Ed.), *Mending the cracks in the ivory tower: Strategies for conflict management in higher education* (pp. 46-59). Boston: Anker.

Sturnick, J. A. (1998). 'And never the twain shall meet': Administrator-faculty conflict. In S. A. Holton (Ed.), *Mending the cracks in the ivory tower: Strategies for conflict management in higher education* (pp. 97-112). Boston: Anker.

Tierney, W. G. (1989). *Curricular landscapes, democratic vistas: Transformative leadership in higher education.* New York: Praeger.

Tierney, W. (1993). *Building communities of difference.* Westport, CT: Bergen & Garvey.

Tierney, W. G., & Rhoads, R. A. (1993). *Enhancing promotion, tenure and beyond (Ashe-Eric Higher Education Reports no. 6).* Washington, DC: George Washington University, School of Education and Human Development.

VanPatten, J. J. (Ed.). (1990). *College teaching and higher education leadership.* Lewiston, NY: Edwin Mellen.

7 Team-Building within HKLS Academic Units

Charles J. Hardy, *Professor and Department Chair, College of Health and Professional Studies, Georgia Southern University*

Frederick K. Whitt, *Professor and Dean, College of Health and Professional Studies, Georgia Southern University*

Teamwork is the essence of life. If there's one thing on which I'm an authority, it's how to blend the talents and strengths of individuals into a force that becomes greater than the sum of its parts. My driving belief is this: great teamwork is the only way to reach our ultimate moments, to create the breakthroughs that define our careers, to fulfill our lives with a sense of lasting significance.

All of us are team players, whether we know it or not. Our significance arrives through our vital connections to other people, through all the teams of our lives....Our best efforts, combined with those of our teammates, grow into something far greater and far more satisfying than anything we could have achieved on our own...

However, teamwork isn't simple. In fact, it can be a frustrating, elusive commodity. That's why there are so many bad teams out there, stuck in neutral or going downhill. Teamwork doesn't appear magically, just because someone mouths the words. It doesn't thrive just because of the presence of talent or ambition. It doesn't flourish simply because a team has tasted success. (Riley, 1993, pp. 15-16)

The concept of TEAM (Together Everyone Achieves More) is that the members of a collective will be more productive working as a team than as individuals. Indeed, it has been said that T-E-A-M-W-O-R-K is how you spell success (Chadwick, 1999). When we join together for a common cause, a sense of team motivates us to greater levels of performance. Orlick (1990) suggested that one of the most gratifying experiences an individual can have is to be a member of a team that works efficiently in a cohesive, task-oriented manner. True teamwork, however, is more than work accomplished by a group of individuals (Salas, 1993). Team members must interact, work toward shared goals, adapt to environmental demands, and balance their individual needs with the needs of the team (Hanson & Lubin, 1988; Salas).

Building an effective team is a formidable task, especially within health, kinesiology, and leisure studies (HKLS) academic units. As Colton (1995) stated, "It is a continuing challenge to administer a group of professionals, all of whom are rugged individualists, not readily amenable to direction or management and eager only to be left alone to carry out their professional and personal pursuits" (p. 326). Yet today, more than ever, the vision of a HKLS professor functioning as an island has been replaced with an expectation that each faculty member be a conscious part of a community, indeed a member of several communities (Stewart, 1995). Thomas Templin (2000), HKLS chair at Purdue University, reinforced this paradigm shift by stating:

> As ego-driven as we all can be, I believe and now have experienced that faculty are willing to balance personal and departmental gain. Individuals are willing to lead or serve on a project team and contribute to the success of a department—of our community. (p. 12)

The extent to which individual HKLS faculty join together to form a community is the defining characteristic of an effective academic unit. It is always a paradox when talent-laden units do not function effectively, while others with less talent and fewer resources develop into highly cohesive performing units. While the basic rationale of a team is to take advantage of the various abilities, backgrounds, and interests of its members, it takes considerable effort to build an effective team. Unfortunately, beyond anecdotal reports on the effectiveness of team-building activities, there is a lack of information on this process in academia, particularly within HKLS departments, schools, and colleges. This chapter presents fundamental team-building processes, components, and recommendations to academic administrators working within HKLS units. It is our hope that the information contained within this chapter will provide the knowledge and activities necessary to "build for your team a feeling of oneness, of dependence upon one another and of strength to be derived by unity" (Vince Lombardi, cited in Anderson, 1990, p. 16).

What Is a Team?

Essentially, a team is any group of people who must interact with each other in order to accomplish shared objectives (Woodcock & Francis, 1981). More specifically, Salas (1993) has defined a team as two or more individuals who must interact interdependently and adaptively to achieve specified, shared, and valued objectives. Moreover, Tannenbaum, Beard, and Salas (1992) argued that members of teams have specific functions to perform. Interdependency of team members and a common goal appear to be the fundamental elements of a team (O'Brien, 1995). From this perspective, it is apparent that HKLS units can be considered teams; therefore, appropriate application of team-building principles is fundamental to success.

What Is an Effective Team?

All teams desire to be effective; however, effectiveness takes on different meanings for different teams (Carron & Hausenblas, 1998). According to Anshel (1994), an effective team is one that consistently and efficiently achieves its goals while maintaining high levels of member satisfaction and loyalty. Hanson and Lubin (1988) proposed that effective teams engage in continuous diagnosis and plan and implement changes based on these diagnoses. Moreover, these authors suggested that effective teams are characterized by an existence of a shared sense of purpose, an understanding of the team's resources, and effective processes. Patten (1981) concluded that healthy organizations are characterized by shared goals and objectives, concern for personal needs and feelings of employees, open communication, and the ability to deal with conflict in an open and constructive manner. Moreover, healthy organizations exhibit a culture of collaboration through mutual respect and trust. Templin (2000) suggested that a supportive culture, frequent interpersonal interaction, and tolerance for personal and professional differences are core characteristics of effective academic departments.

Teams are constantly developing and changing as they respond to both internal and external factors. These changes may be barely noticeable or may cause significant upheaval and adaptation. Tuckman (1965) and Tuckman and Jensen (1977) suggested that in order to understand the dynamics of a team, we must understand the stages of development that occur in groups throughout their life cycle. These authors delineated five distinct stages: forming, storming, norming, performing, and adjourning. In the forming stage, the group engages in orientating behaviors, defining objectives, getting acquainted with each other, and establishing boundaries. This is thought to be an anxious period, with members assessing each other and the group as a whole.

The storming stage represents a period of conflict and internal stress. Team unity is challenged as individual members attempt to stand on their own and highlight their unique qualities. This is often a very emotional period, with anxieties about how individual roles fit within the team being paramount. During this stage, leaders should attempt to reduce uncertainty by clearly communicating individual responsibilities and demonstrating how individual contributions facilitate the development of the team. The quiet following the storm is referred to as the norming stage. A sense of unity, togetherness, and effectiveness emerges during this stage, and the leader should focus on encouraging individuals to offer social as well as task-related support to teammates. In the performing stage, the team focuses on accomplishing its goals and objectives. Team members have moved beyond what Templin (2000) called "superficial colleagueship" and have formed into a functioning team with a shared sense of purpose. Moreover, the team becomes a "place of pride, identification, support, and camaraderie" (Templin, p. 12). The final stage, adjourning, involves adjustment to termination of the team or the disengagement of teammates. According to Danish, Owens, Green, and Brunelle (1997), team members experience a sense of loss and/or anxiety during this stage. With academic teams, this stage is brought about by retirements, resignations, non-renewals, or faculty burnout.

Recently, Covey (1997) suggested that effective families experience various phases as they move from a survival focus to a significance focus. For one thing, there is shift in thinking from problem-solving to creating. This change in mindset leads to a completely different "culture." Covey describes this positive team culture:

> *It's like the difference between feeling exhausted from morning until night and feeling rested, energized, and enthused. Instead of feeling frustrated, mired in concerns, and surrounded by dark clouds of despair, you feel optimistic, invigorated, and full of hope. You're filled with positive energy that leads to a creative, synergistic mode. Focused on your vision, you take problems in stride. (pp. 322-323)*

How Does a Team Develop?

The Team-Building Process

Team-building has been one of the most enduring themes in the organizational development literature (Beer, 1976; Buller, 1986; DeMeuse & Liebowitz, 1981; Tannenbaum et al., 1992; Woodman & Sherwood, 1980). Hardy and Crace (1997) argued that team-building is best viewed as a team intervention that enhances performance by positively affecting team processes or synergy. Team synergy can be defined as "the interaction of two or more agents or forces so that the combined effort is far greater than the sum of their individual efforts" (Mears & Voehl, 1994, p. 4). Beer indicated that team-building interventions can take four different approaches: (1) goal-setting, (2) interpersonal relations, (3) role expectations, and (4) concern for production and people. In actuality, however, it is rare that team-building interventions rely on only one approach.

The goal of any such intervention is to increase the effectiveness of the group by enhancing its tendency to remain united in the pursuit of its goals (Carron, 1982; Carron, Spink, & Prapavessis, 1997). Cohesion is thought to have both task and social dimensions, and team-building interventions typically involve a range of strategies that are designed to enhance one or both of these dimensions (Smith & Smoll, 1997). Research on the effectiveness of this notion has indicated that there is a positive relationship between cohesion and team success (Widmeyer, Carron, & Brawley, 1993). Moreover, studies have demonstrated positive relations between cohesion and the degree of satisfaction derived by individuals from membership on teams (Williams & Hacker, 1982).

Several writers (e.g., Carron & Hausenblas, 1998; Woodcock & Francis, 1981) have indicated that effective team-building results in a productive work group that possesses six characteristics: (1) team leadership is coherent, visionary, and acceptable, (2) team members understand and accept their roles and responsibilities, (3) members dedicate their efforts to collective achievement, (4) climate is positive, energetic, and empowering, (5) team meetings are efficient in terms of time and resources, and (6) weaknesses in team capability are diagnosed and reduced or eliminated.

Tannenbaum et al. (1992) argued that team-building can be targeted to "improve team processes, enhance individual or team characteristics, or modify the work structure of the task" (p. 122). According to their model, team effectiveness is best understood from an input, output, and "throughput" perspective. Team inputs include individual and team characteristics, the characteristics of the task on which the team is working, and the manner in which the work is structured. The outputs represent individual and team changes as well as team performance. Teams use output feedback to modify the input variables. "Throughputs" are the processes by which the team converts the inputs into outputs. From this perspective, team-building can have both a direct and indirect influence on team processes. For example, team-building can directly affect such processes as coordination of resources, interpersonal communication, problem-solving, and decision-making. Team-building can also affect the team indirectly, through various input variables (e.g., team cohesiveness).

Team-building is needed when the lack of effective teamwork is a serious barrier to effective performance. More specifically, team-building is needed when some or all of the following symptoms are present: (1) low productivity, (2) unresolved interpersonal conflicts, (3) inappropriate use of individual resources, (4) unclear discussions, (5) role ambiguity, (6) a general lack of interest and creativity, and (7) complaints that the team does not respond to the needs of others or meet its responsibilities (Hanson & Lubin, 1988).

Team-building within HKLS units is not a one-shot intervention or "quick fix" that can create cohesiveness and productivity. To be effective, it must be an ongoing process that complements the developmental level of the team. While it is important to understand and respect contextual variability within and among different departments, schools, colleges, and institutions, effective team-building in any HKLS unit should include five core components.

First, a diagnosis of the team must be conducted. Based on the work of Brawley and Paskevich (1997), descriptive information should be gathered regarding four main factors: (1) characteristics of the unit and its members, (2) the purpose and functions of the unit, (3) the physical environment in which the unit operates, and (4) the unit's perception of itself and its interpersonal and group dynamics. Further, these authors suggested that questions be developed concerning the effects of group size, the potential social process losses, the group's stage of development and level of cohesion, and the potential barriers to team-building interventions.

One effective and practical approach to gathering pertinent data for team diagnosis involves the use of the Life Values Inventory (LVI) (Crace & Brown, 2000). The LVI measures 14 life-values: achievement, belonging, concern for the environment, concern for others, creativity, financial prosperity, health and activity, humility, independence, interdependence, objective analysis, privacy, responsibility, and spirituality. Faculty can use the LVI to crystallize and prioritize their values and then share these value structures with fellow team members. This approach can also be helpful in determining areas of congruence between importance and action, as well as sources of stress and hot-button issues for individuals and the team. These activities often enhance understanding and foster mutual respect, which are the cornerstones of the team-building process.

Crace and Hardy (1997) argued that since behavior is a manifestation of values, it is much harder to manipulate a desired values profile without it being noticed by other team members. Indeed, it is not unusual for colleagues to nod their heads in agreement when an individual faculty member discloses his or her values profile, or to question values that an individual deems important but does not exhibit in his or her behavior. Nor is it unusual for both intra- and interpersonal conflicts to be more fully understood through the clarification of value structures. Faculty and administrators should be on the lookout for intra-role, inter-role, and intrapersonal conflicts. Intra-role conflicts occur whenever the demands of the job conflict with the values of the individual. Faculty who value independence and find the work environment controlling will experience this kind of conflict. Inter-role conflicts occur whenever the demands of the job preclude individuals from satisfying values related to other parts of their life, or when other life roles preclude them from satisfying important work values. Finally, intrapersonal conflicts are experienced when an individual holds two contradictory values to be important, such as independence and belonging. Once faculty and administrators identify the values-based conflicts underlying their stress, appropriate management and intervention strategies can be implemented at both the individual and unit levels.

Effective Team-Building in HKLS

Factors that promote or interfere with team cohesion can also be identified, and team-building action plans can be developed and implemented.

The values-based approach to team-building has been most useful with HKLS units; after all, values guide behavior, form the basis for goal-setting and motivation, and serve as standards to evaluate behavior (Rokeach, 1973). Values are developed so that individuals can meet their needs in socially accepted ways, and they tend to be more central determinants of behavior than interests, preferences, and attitudes. Crace and Hardy (1997) maintained that a focus on values reveals a more in-depth understanding of an individual's motivation and of the forces that drive teams. Moreover, values clarification can help identify causes of, and solutions to, individual and team conflicts. Such an approach provides a much deeper approach to team-building that is typically experienced. Crace and Hardy suggested that by focusing on this more fundamental determinant of behavior, faculty and administrators can get to the root of the "why" underlying certain team behaviors.

Once individual value systems have been identified and discussed, a team-values profile (Team V) can be developed. An example of a "Team V" for a HKLS department is as follows:

- *Responsibility*—it is important for us to be dependable and trustworthy
- *Concern for Others*—the well-being of others is important
- *Achievement*—it is important to challenge ourselves and to work hard to improve
- *Health and Activity*—it is important to be healthy and physically active
- *Interdependence*—it is important to follow the traditions and expectations of the department, college, and university.

Once the Team V has been developed, the team can examine its strengths and weaknesses. Moreover, individuals can discuss similarities and differences between their personal values profile and the team's (Crace & Brown, 1997).

Unlike the majority of team-building models that focus on the team itself, the values-based approach places an emphasis on understanding and respecting the "I" in team. We have also found that the effectiveness of the model is dependent on the facilitator's experience and training in areas such as assessment, group dynamics, human-resource development, and performance psychology. Thus, while you can determine the role of the "I" in team on your own, we suggest that you let go of your role and rely on an objective professional who is trained in team-building. For a more in-depth presentation of the values-based model of team-building, see Crace and Hardy (1997).

Once the diagnosis is complete, it is important to develop a shared vision. That is, the team must address the question, "Who do we want to become?" It is important to use the data gained in the diagnostic phase as a touchstone when developing this unity of purpose. Yukelson (1997) indicated that team-building starts with the leader sharing a vision of "what can be" if everyone pulls together for the sake of the team. This is similar to Covey's (1997) notion that effective families are "proactive" units ("Habit 1") that "begin with the end in mind" ("Habit 2"). The team's vision statement must paint a picture of a desired state of being; it should be clear, concise, and inspirational. A mission statement should indicate the purpose of your team, including who you are, what you do, how you do it, and whom you serve. Chadwick (1999) maintained that leaders should read aloud the vision and mission statements every 28 days so that the team is constantly focused on who they are and where they are headed. In this light, we suggest that the vision and mission statements be made public. Place these statements on bulletin boards and the department web page, and send them along with an e-mail each month to all members of the team. Perhaps the most important aspect, however, is to ensure that all members of the team have input into the development of the vision and mission of the unit. Developing these statements takes time, so take the time! Once your vision and mission are set, all the other pieces of the team-building puzzle will fall into place.

Team goals must be developed for achieving the vision. This component addresses the question, "How do we get there?" Team goals have been shown to facilitate both cohesion and performance (Widmeyer & Ducharme, 1997), largely by: (1) directing attention, (2) increasing task effort, (3) increasing task persistence, and (4) motivating the development of suitable task strategies (Carron, 1993). Moreover, Carron asserts that role clarity and acceptance are improved through effective team goal-setting as well. This is similar to Covey's (1997) notion that effective families "put first things first" ("Habit 3").

In their goal-setting program for teams, Widmeyer and Ducharme (1997) suggested the following principles: (1) establish long-term goals first, (2) establish clear paths to the long-term goals, (3) involve all team members in establishing goals, (4) monitor progress toward team goals, (5) give rewards for such progress, and (6) foster collective efficacy concerning team-goal attainment. Furthermore, as with the vision statement, team goals should be made public. Department goals can be posted in the main office and in each member's office. Leaders should refer to the team's progress toward the goals at least once each term.

We have used a model that includes the development of a university-wide strategic plan and of college, departmental, and individual goals. Our university's strategic plan represents a long-term (5-to-10-year) focus on what the university—and therefore each college and department—desires to become. Six strategic themes provide the structure to achieve this vision: academic distinction, student-centeredness, technological advances, transcultural opportunities, private-public partnerships, and enhancement of the physical environment. On an annual basis, departments can form theme clusters (groups of faculty) to generate team goals for each theme. Such an activity has been shown to be very effective in promoting commitment to the team's goals and making sure that the unit stays connected to the larger university agenda. This approach can also be extended to individual faculty, ensuring that their goals are connected to the department's. For this to happen, department goals must reflect the diversity of the group. An annual performance review can be used as both a "navigational" correction for the department and an incentive for individual contributions to the team.

It is important to remember that there is a complex relationship between individual and group goal-setting. Zander (1971) identified the following factors in this relationship: (1) an individual's goals for self, (2) an individual's goals for the group, (3) the group's goals, and (4) the group's goals for the individual. Widmeyer and Ducharme (1997) suggested that each of these goal relations must be considered when one is designing team-building strategies. Goals should also be "S-M-A-R-T"—that is, specific, measurable, attainable, realistic, and time-bound (Weinberg & Gould, 1999). Moreover, we argue that goals should be consistent with the "Team V" and the department's shared vision.

Principles that guide the unit's behavior must be developed and agreed upon. Several writers have emphasized that team unity and synergistic empowerment can be created through the development of shared principles (Covey, 1989, 1997; DePree, 1989; Riley, 1993; Templin, 2000; Yukelson, 1997). Riley maintained that having individuals enact the core values of the team by reinforcing appropriate team-oriented behaviors can be a very powerful form of team-building. Dean Smith, former men's basketball coach at the University of North Carolina, is renowned in coaching circles for his commitment to team principles. His "Carolina System" was based on the guiding principles of "playing hard, playing smart, and playing together." These principles were underscored by Smith's own core values (putting people above all else; requiring that the individual talents of players be subordinate to the good of the team; leading with conviction, care, and character) (Chadwick, 1999). Being committed to principles comes with its share of stress, however. For example, in an attempt to demean coach Smith's belief that the team is more important than the individual, some critics joked that he was the only person ever to hold Michael Jordan—his most famous player—to fewer than 20 points in a game (Chadwick, 1999).

One particularly good principle is Covey's (1997) "Think win-win" ("Habit 4"). This principle places relationships first; "it's the underlying motive, the nurturing attitude out of which understanding and synergy grow" (p. 171). Along with two of his other principles—"Seek first to understand, then to be understood" ("Habit 5") and "Synergize" ("Habit 6")—this principle leads to enhanced "social weather" (p. 171) inside the team. That is, exercising these principles leads to the creation of an environment characterized by respect, understanding, and creative cooperation rather than self-focus and interpersonal competition.

An excellent example of using guiding principles in the team-building process within a HKLS department is presented by Templin (2000). During Templin's attempt to renew and change his department, the following principles were agreed upon by the faculty: "(a) change should be geared toward quality improvement and the elimination of redundancy and inefficiency, (b) change calls for leadership and active participation, (c) change calls call for community building, erasing fragmentation, and building partnerships and bridges, (d) change calls for continuous evaluation and adjustments, and (e) change calls for communication—believing and trusting one another, having respect, encouraging openness, and achieving collegiality" (p. 13). We have found it useful to develop two sets of guiding principles. One set—centrality, quality, viability, and comparative advantage—is for program development and reviews. The other set—grace, respect, wisdom, and passion—provides guidance on intra- and interpersonal issues.

Finally, an effective team culture must be established and nurtured. Team culture is multidimensional, and its development is dependent on a wide variety of factors. These include, but are not limited to, similarity, commitment, role clarification, and communication. Similarity in attitudes, aspirations, commitments, and ability is important in any department (Carron, 1993). Remember, however, that the more diverse a group is, the greater its potential. Thus, while we are not advocating homogeneity in personality, ethnicity, race, or socioeconomic status, we do believe that all members of a unit need to be on the same page in terms of individual and team expectations. Moreover, since conflict is natural in a dynamic and diverse group, conflict management must be an important aspect of the team culture.

Team norms reflect a consensus about behaviors that are acceptable. An effective unit must establish a norm for productivity as well as for how people are expected to interact with one another. If such an approach is to positively affect the culture of the unit, members of the unit must be willing to compromise and sacrifice for the common good. It should also be noted that administrators must be willing to reinforce such sacrifices with merit pay and during tenure and promotion reviews and decisions.

Research has demonstrated that when individuals understand their roles (role clarity), accept their roles (role acceptance), and perform their roles to the best of their capabilities (role performance), a positive, cohesive, and task-focused climate is developed and maintained (Carron, 1993). The roles that individuals are expected to perform within the unit should be clearly articulated and made known to all team members. Moreover, it is important to reinforce on a consistent basis the importance of all roles in relation to the unit's success. Carron (1993) argued that when individuals perceive the importance of their roles and responsibilities to the collective, they are more willing to carry them out.

Effective communication is also important in establishing and maintaining a functional team culture. According to Yukelson (1993), team-building requires a group climate of openness. The more open individual members of the unit can be, the better their chances of developing into a cohesive, productive team: "Harmony grows when you really listen to others and they listen to you, when you are considerate of their feelings and they are considerate of yours, when you accept their differences and they accept yours, and when you help them and they help you" (Orlick, 1986, p. 143).

One aspect of improving communication that is consistently overlooked by most faculty and administrators is effective listening. Listening has consistently been found to be one of the most important characteristics of effective organizations (Burke, 1997). Rosenfeld, Wilder, Crace, and Hardy (1990) suggested that active listening—where the listener is attentive and engaged in the listening process—is fundamental to effective communication.

Chairs and deans in HKLS spend quite a bit of time providing feedback to individuals and groups of faculty. To ensure that feedback is effective, Smith, Smoll, and Curtis (1977) have suggested the use of the "sandwich" approach, wherein positive statements surround corrective and constructive feedback. Feedback given through this approach can enhance the self-esteem of individuals as well as prevent conflict.

Nonverbal communication is also a critical aspect of nurturing an effective team climate (Burke, 1997). The key element here is to ensure that one's message is compatible with the manner in which it is delivered. When nonverbal and verbal behaviors are consistent, communication is enhanced because the possibility of mixed messages is decreased. Yukelson (1993) argued that interpersonal respect is often communicated through nonverbal channels. Remember, "actions speak louder than words."

In order to improve communication, it is also important to develop a foundation of interpersonal trust (Burke, 1997). Trust may develop from working together through different challenges over time. However, it may also be necessary to focus some extra energy on establishing trust. For example, special activities and challenges can be designed to help unit members learn to trust one another. To develop trust between administrators and faculty, both parties need to be honest, open, fair, and consistent with one another so that each can know what to expect. If the "P" word is used, promises must be kept. Problems emerge when "hidden agendas" are perceived. Consistency helps to provide confidence and security in a relationship (Anshel, 1994). Faculty need to have an idea of how administrators will respond in varying situations; as Burke maintained, mixed messages cause "mixed-up" relationships.

Finally, nurturing a team culture includes renewal activities that energize or "sharpen the saw" ("Habit 7") for both individuals and the team (Covey, 1997). Covey maintains that it is important for families to engage in physical, social, mental, and spiritual renewal in order to enhance their quality of life. Similarly, when these activities are experienced within a team, relationships are enhanced. For example, unit members who exercise together increase not only their physical fitness, but also their social ties.

Traditions emerge from repeated renewal activities (Covey, 1997). These can range from purely social events to academic endeavors such as distinguished lectures, honor days, and faculty debates. Somewhere in between are faculty retreats, where faculty get away from campus and focus on a wide range of topics. One example of a simple yet effective renewal activity is to set aside a time when faculty meet in a lounge for treats, java, and fellowship. We find this to be a very enjoyable and regenerating experience. One important rule is that no "shop talk" should be allowed. This is a time to simply enjoy each other's company and "sharpen the saw." There are many traditions that can be fostered through such events. The key factor is to provide activities in which members of the unit can have fun, be energized, and enjoy some high-quality time with one another.

Recommendations for Department Chairs and Deans

As with any type of leader, chairs and deans must integrate faculty into effective units that perform with a sense of pride, excellence, and collective identity. The following represent recommendations for chairs and deans looking to accomplish this objective. These recommendations are based on the core components of team-building as well as on our own experiences in team-building with both departments and colleges. Not all recommendations will work in every situation. It is up to you to determine the efficacy of a specific recommendation in building your team.

Commit to building your team. Orlick (1986) stated that "the most important thing you can do to increase team harmony is to make a commitment to do so" (p. 98). Believe in the team and the team-building process and engage in team-building activities. It is not enough to "talk the walk"; you must also "walk the talk." If you are going to talk about being a team, do all you can do to establish a team culture. We have found that organizing special workshops and/or retreats (or, rather, "advances") away from campus provides a unique opportunity to demonstrate your commitment to the team-building process. We have also found that developing a mentoring system within your unit demonstrates a similar commitment. This is particularly important for new faculty. Such a system can be informal or formal, personal and professional, and can involve faculty from within and outside the unit. Everyone has something to offer, so all members of the team should be encouraged to both mentor and seek mentoring. We have also found that having frequent renewal and perspective-building activities provides opportunities for faculty to recharge their batteries. Faculty-appreciation days, recreation outings, pot-luck luncheons, faculty picnics, and community-service activities are just a few examples. This is particularly important during times of conflict. Be creative, and have members of the team assist with this process so that a healthy perspective can be found and the current challenge can be successfully negotiated. Remember, the key with these activities is to make sure that the team understands the benefit of such experiences: no one benefits from forced social interaction.

Get to know the "I" in "TEAM." Use the LVI to assess individual and team values. This instrument and the values-based model presented earlier will result in mutual understanding and respect. This is particularly important in environments where an "us versus them" mentality exists between faculty members or between the faculty and the administration. Moreover, understanding and respecting individuals with different value systems facilitates the strength-in-diversity ethos within the academy.

Develop a vision, a mission, and guiding principles. Leaders of character have the ability to unite individuals into an effective team. Unity of purpose distinguishes exceptional units from average ones. Guiding principles ensure that the process is as important as the product. Chairs and deans must take a leading role in telling their unit's "story" once it is developed. Stephen Portch, the Chancellor of Georgia's university system, suggested that HKLS professionals must tell their story by "capturing attention, sketching pictures, and touching humanity" (Portch, 1999).

Develop team goals. A department or college without goals is doomed to failure. To be effective, you have to plan your work and then work your plan. It is important that the team develop goals. Individual ownership of these goals is a must. Individual and team values should serve as touchstones for team goals, since goals will only be effective if they are based on explicit value systems. Remember to encourage individuals to make their personal goals congruent with the team goals. It is also important to hold individuals accountable for team success and failure.

Communicate effectively. Communication for HKLS chairs and deans involves many facets, including daily one-on-one interactions with faculty and staff, distribution of information, departmental meetings, and more formal conferences and meetings. Developing newsletters, setting up electronic listservs and chat rooms, and initiating advisory councils composed of faculty, staff, students, and community members are all examples of effective communication techniques for academic units. Remember that no single communication style or technique will meet all needs. Respect individual differences and actively listen for both content and emotion. Make sure that you are timely, accurate, systematic, and consistent in your communication. Conflict is inevitable, even for those of us who are excellent communicators. During periods of conflict, always remember to take the high road: avoid gossiping about and backstabbing members of your team. We have found that when we clearly articulate responsibilities, conflict is reduced. When individuals have high role clarity and role acceptance, role performance is enhanced. All communication should instill an attitude of "same goal, different roles" (Corbin, 1991). When you must take action to manage conflict, stay focused on the problem and seek win-win solutions. When you are angry, it helps to pause before responding. Responses based on strong, negative emotions are not effective team-building behaviors.

Continually build your team. It is important to embrace a continuous improvement model for your HKLS unit. Any good gardener will tell you that it is not enough to simply plant the seeds; you must constantly water, fertilize, weed, and prune. Similarly, HKLS faculty need to be reinforced, supported, redirected, mentored, and facilitated if the team is to grow and develop. Team-building requires an enormous amount of energy. We often joke with each other that team-building within HKLS units is like "putting beads on a string without a knot at the end." That is, your work as the leader of the team is never done. Team-building is an important part of developing into an effective HKLS administrator. While it may be time-consuming and involve a great deal of planning, the rewards that result from investing in the team-building process will significantly enhance both the internal functioning and external perception of your unit.

Summary

We have enjoyed sharing our ideas about the team-building process within academia. It is our hope that this chapter will provide the fundamentals of team-building while at the same time serving as a catalyst for increased attention on this most important process. The techniques presented in this chapter are only the basic tools and, in some cases, are based on the art rather than the science of team-building. The tools are not ends in themselves, nor are they exclusive to the academic context. However, we hope that the information presented here will help those who face the tremendous challenge of unifying a collection of individuals into an effective team. The value of this chapter will be determined by its ability to serve as a foundational resource for HKLS administrators looking to enhance their units. We hope that you will build on our thoughts. We firmly believe that the future well-being of the academy will depend on the development of a team culture.

Riley (1993) maintained that the most difficult thing for individuals to do when they are part of a team is to resist the "Disease of Me." While there is no single cure for this "disease," team-building interventions can help faculty work together in an attempt to achieve their unit's potential. It bears repeating—teamwork is more than just work accomplished by a group of individuals (Salas, 1993).

When you see geese heading for the winter, flying in a "V" formation, think about what science has learned about why they fly that way. As each bird flaps its wings, it creates uplift for the bird immediately following it. By flying in a "V" formation, the whole flock can fly at least 71 percent farther than if each bird flew on its own. Perhaps people who share a common direction can get where they are going quicker and easier if they cooperate.

Whenever, a goose falls out of formation, it feels the resistance of trying to go it alone and quickly gets back into functioning to take advantage of flying with the flock. If we have as much sense as a goose, we will work with others who are going the same way as we are. When the lead goose gets tired, he rotates back in the wing and another goose flies on the point. It pays to take turns doing hard jobs from our group. Perhaps the geese honking from behind are even the 'cheering squad' to encourage those up front to keep up their speed.

Finally, if a goose weakens or is wounded and falls out of formation, two geese fall out and follow him down to help and protect him. They stay with him until he is either able to fly or until he is dead. Then they set out on their own, or with another formation, until they catch up with their group. If we had [the] sense of a goose, we would stand by each other like that. (Mears & Voehl, 1994, p. 2)

Team effectiveness is dependent on the development and nurturing of a team culture, and team-building can assist with this development. Successful team-building interventions require: a culture that supports a team approach; teams that are receptive and prepared to undertake the process; resources to aid the process; and leaders who are aware of the "building blocks" of effective teamwork. For team-building to succeed, however, all team members must invest in the process. The components presented in this chapter represent a framework that chairs and deans can use to accomplish this goal. Depending on the team and the situation the team finds itself in, different core components of team-building will need to be emphasized. Ultimately, chairs and deans are responsible for developing team chemistry. In addition to creating harmony within the unit, they must also blend the talents of individual faculty into an effective team that performs with a sense of pride, enthusiasm, and collective identity (Yukelson, 1997). Ultimately, the leadership skills of chairs and deans play a vital role in the effectiveness of the team-building process.

About the Authors

Charles J. Hardy, professor and chair, Health and Kinesiology, Georgia Southern University, is in his seventh year as a department chair. He has consulted with many academic, athletic, and business "teams" on the team-building process.

Frederick K. Whitt, professor and dean, College of Health and Professional Studies, Georgia Southern University, has 25 years experience in higher education, nine years as a dean and eight years as a department chair. In addition, he has implemented and directed leadership-development activities within campus and community environments.

References

Anderson, P. (1990). *Great quotes from great leaders*. Lombard, IL: Celebrating Excellence.

Anshel, M. H. (1994). *Sport psychology: From theory to practice* (2nd ed.). Scottsdale, AZ: Gorsuch Scarisbrick.

Beer, M. (1976). The technology of organization development. In M. D. Dunnette (Ed.), *Handbook of industrial and organizational psychology* (pp. 937-994). Chicago: Rand McNally.

Brawley, L. R., & Paskevich, D. M. (1997). Conducting team-building research in the context of sport and exercise. *Journal of Applied Sport Psychology, 9*, 11-40.

Buller, P. F. (1986). The team-building/task-performance relation: Some conceptual and methodological refinements. *Group and Organization Studies, 11*, 147-168.

Burke, K. L. (1997). Communication in sports: Research and practice. *Journal of Interdisciplinary Research in Physical Education, 2*(1), 39-52.

Carron, A. V. (1982). Cohesiveness in sport groups: Interpretations and considerations. *Journal of Sport Psychology, 4*, 123-138.

Carron, A. V. (1993). The sport team as an effective group. In J. Williams (Ed.), *Applied sport psychology: Personal growth to peak performance* (2nd ed.) (pp. 110-121). Mountain View, CA: Mayfield.

Carron, A. V., & Hausenblas, H. A. (1998). *Group dynamics in sport* (2nd ed.). Morgantown, WV: Fitness Information Technology.

Carron, A. V., Spink, K. S., & Prapavessis, H. (1997). Team-building and cohesiveness in the sport and exercise setting: Use of indirect interventions. *Journal of Applied Sport Psychology, 9*, 61-72.

Chadwick, D. (1999). *The 12 leadership principles of Dean Smith.* New York: Total Sports Illustrated.

Colton, J. (1995). The role of the department in the groves of academe. In A. L. Deneff & C. D. Goodwin (Eds.), *The academic handbook* (2nd ed.) (pp. 315-333). Durham, NC: Duke University Press.

Corbin, C. B. (1991). Further reactions to Newell: Becoming a field is more important than saying we are one. *Quest, 43*, 224-229.

Covey, S. R. (1989). *The seven habits of highly effective people.* New York: Fireside.

Covey, S. R. (1997). *The seven habits of highly effective families.* New York: St. Martin's.

Crace, R. K., & Brown, D. (1997). *Building effective teams.* Chapel Hill, NC: Life Values Resources.

Crace, R. K., & Brown, D. (2000). *Life Values Inventory.* Chapel Hill, NC: Life Values Resources.

Crace, R. K., & Hardy, C. J. (1997). Individual values and the team-building process. *Journal of Applied Sport Psychology, 9*, 41-60.

Danish, S. J., Owens, S. S., Green, S., & Brunelle, J. P. (1997). Building bridges for disengagement: The transition process for individuals and teams. *Journal of Applied Sport Psychology, 9*, 154-167.

DeMeuse, K. P., & Liebowitz, S. J. (1981). An empirical analysis of team-building research. *Group and Organization Studies, 6*, 357-378.

DePree, M. (1989). *Leadership is an art.* New York: Doubleday.

Hanson, P. G., & Lubin, B. (1988). Team-building as group development. In W. B. Reddy & K. Jamison (Eds.), *Team-building: Blueprints for productivity and satisfaction* (pp. 76-78). Alexandria, VA: National Institute for Applied Behavioral Science.

Hardy, C. J., & Crace, R. K. (1997). Introduction to the team-building primer. *Journal of Applied Sport Psychology, 9*, 1-10.

Mears, P., & Voehl, F. (1994). *Team-building: A structured learning approach.* Delray Beach, FL: St. Lucie.

O'Brien, M. (1995). *Who's got the ball? And other nagging questions about team life.* San Francisco: Jossey-Bass.

Orlick, T. (1986). *Psyching for sport.* Champaign, IL: Human Kinetics.

Orlick, T. (1990). *In pursuit of excellence* (2nd ed.). Champaign, IL: Leisure.

Patten, T. H. (1981). *Organizational development through team-building.* New York: John Wiley & Sons.

Portch, S. (1999). The toughest teaching: Capturing attention, sketching pictures, and touching humanity. *Quest, 51,* 94-101.

Riley, P. (1993). *The winner within: A life plan for team players.* New York: G. P. Putnam's Sons.

Rokeach, M. (1973). *The nature of human values.* New York: Free Press.

Rosenfeld, L., Wilder, L., Crace, R. K., & Hardy, C. J. (1990). Communication fundamentals: Active listening. *Sport Psychology Training Bulletin, 1*(5), 1-8.

Salas, E. (1993). Team training and performance. *Science Agenda, 6*(1), 9-11.

Smith, R. E., Smoll, F. L., & Curtis, B. (1977). Coaching roles and relationships. In J. R. Thomas (Ed.), *Youth sport guide for parents and coaches* (pp. 7-23). Reston, VA: American Alliance for Health, Physical Education, Recreation, and Dance.

Smith, R. E., & Smoll, F. L. (1997). Coach-mediated team-building in youth sports. *Journal of Applied Sport Psychology, 9,* 114-132.

Stewart, P. (1995). The academic community. In A. L Deneff & C. D. Goodwin (Eds.), *The academic handbook* (2nd ed.) (pp. 334-340). Durham, NC: Duke University Press.

Tannenbaum, S. I., Beard, R. L., & Salas, E. (1992). Team-building and its influence on team effectiveness: An examination of conceptual and empirical developments. In K. Kelley (Ed.), *Issues, theory, and research in industrial/organizational psychology* (pp. 117-153). Amsterdam: Elsevier.

Templin, T. (2000). Department renewal: Reflections on the induction period of a new department head. *The Chronicle of Physical Education in Higher Education, 11*(2), 11-14.

Tuckman, B. W. (1965). Developmental sequence in small groups. *Psychological Bulletin, 63,* 384-399.

Tuckman, B. W., & Jensen, M. C. (1977). Stages of small-group development revisited. *Group and Organizational Studies, 2,* 419-427.

Weinberg, R. S., & Gould, D. (1999). *Foundations of sport and exercise psychology* (2nd ed.). Champaign, IL: Human Kinetics.

Widmeyer, W. N., Carron, A. V., & Brawley, L. R. (1993). Group cohesion in sport and exercise. In R. N. Singer, M. Murphey, & L. K. Tennant (Eds.), *Handbook of research on sport psychology* (pp. 672-692). New York: Macmillan.

Widmeyer, W. N., & Ducharme, K. (1997). Team-building through team goal setting. *Journal of Applied Sport Psychology, 9,* 97-113.

Williams, J. M., & Hacker, C. M. (1982). Causal relationships among cohesion, satisfaction, and performance in women's intercollegiate field hockey teams. *Journal of Sport Psychology, 4,* 324-337.

Woodcock, M., & Francis, D. (1981). *Organization development through team-building.* New York: John Wiley & Sons.

Woodman, R. W., & Sherwood, J. J. (1980). The role of team development in organizational effectiveness: A critical review. *Psychological Bulletin, 88,* 166-186.

Yukelson, D. (1993). Communicating effectively. In J. Williams (Ed.), *Applied sport psychology: Personal growth to peak performance* (2nd ed.) (pp. 122-136). Mountain View, CA: Mayfield.

Yukelson, D. (1997). Principles of effective team-building interventions in sport: A direct services approach at Penn State University. *Journal of Applied Sport Psychology, 9,* 73-96.

Zander, A. (1971). *Motives and goals in groups.* New York: Academic.

8 Leading Faculty and Staff through a Changing Higher-Education Matrix

Ronald S. Feingold, *Chair, Department of Health Studies, Physical Education, and Human Performance Science, Adelphi University*

"Details, Details, Details" – Administrators need to attend to details.
⊶ Ronald S. Feingold

Leading faculty and staff through a shifting higher-education matrix—where course workloads, central administration, and department and university missions are all subject to change—is a complex endeavor that requires insight, wisdom, creativity, patience, and perseverance. Finding all of these traits perfected in one person is difficult; thus, administrators in higher education may be better off sharing their responsibilities with others. New directions and priorities established within an academic institution may influence faculty in a number of ways, affecting their teaching, their definitions of service, and their scholarly standards. Both tenured and untenured faculty may with good cause fear the effects of these changes and become insecure.

Being an administrator in an academic unit is a very different job than that of an administrator in a business setting. In an academic setting, administrators must provide an environment that will promote change, vitality, scholarship, service, and commitment to students. The majority of the individuals being managed have lifetime contracts; have more knowledge about their area of specialization than the administrator; and have little financial incentive for doing an exceptional jobs, and few disincentives to perform below par. This is quite different from being able to lead and motivate individuals in the business sector, where one can provide financial incentives and where employee contracts are often short-term.

One may view change as a threat to one's job security, sense of control, and comfort level. On the other hand, one may view change as an opportunity for leadership, greater control, and enhanced comfort. In this chapter, the reader will be exposed to administrative applications and theories that may provide valuable information on gaining support and commitment from faculty, central administrators, and community members. A variety of themes will be touched upon as a process is established for leading faculty and staff through the ever-changing education matrix.

Fostering Passion and Commitment

Chairs and deans are responsible for academic units, but it is also extremely important for them to become involved in the university beyond the unit. In particular, they should participate in or chair important committees (admissions, academic affairs, tenure and promotion, presidential task forces) and, eventually, join the university senate. While on these committees, administrators have an opportunity to network with other faculty leaders and gain their respect. They also have the opportunity to recommend faculty from their unit to important committees. Each time one of your faculty members interacts in a positive way with members of other units, it can enhance the credibility of your unit and lead to collaborative projects and curricular development.

In addition to involvement within the university, a passion for the profession oftentimes leads one into the community and various professional affiliations. Again, a good leader is able to bring both young and experienced faculty into these expanded roles. During one of my own recent involvements—as an advisor to a middle-school wellness program—I was able to coax an experienced social scientist from my department to evaluate the effectiveness of the program. Through my longstanding involvement with the Long Island chapter of the American Heart Association (as a board member and chair), many of the exercise-science faculty have become acquainted with the association's Exercise Committee and with many medical and hospital administration personnel. Through my involvement with a local hospital, these same faculty have developed cooperative workshops and in-service training programs for hospital workers. Many of the faculty have also followed my involvement with the American Alliance for Health, Physical Education, Recreation, and Dance (AAHPERD) and have taken on important leadership positions in state and district associations. Similarly, I have fostered faculty involvement in the National Association for Physical Education in Higher Education (NAPEHE), Physical Best, and AIESEP (International Association for Physical Education in Higher Education). Another recent project involved a joint committee of sports-management faculty, business faculty, and school teachers in the production and development of new curricula in sports management and sports marketing for high schools. Other projects in which faculty have become involved include: a youth-sports workshop with local Little League leadership; an American Heart Association workshop for teachers on the implementation of fitness- and nutrition-education programs; and the development of aging programs with the help of faculty specializing in social work, health, nursing, and exercise science.

In each case, the projects helped faculty collaborate with community members, applied clinicians, practitioners, and faculty in other disciplines. Besides enhancing respect for one another by working on societal problems related to our profession, faculty can gain a more holistic perspective and an appreciation for "real-world" applications by participating in such projects. These expanded experiences can significantly help faculty relate to their students and present information that is more relevant to them. Their involvement also helps in the recruitment of students and in the enhancement of the department's reputation within the community and among practitioners in various fields. Outreach projects can motivate faculty to become committed to the belief that our disciplines are critically important to people of all ages—that we can make a difference in what happens in schools, communities, society, and the profession. Such passion, commitment, and involvement should be supported by the unit administrator so that faculty will come to view their involvement on broader projects as being more important than their own personal interests.

Faculty with expertise in a particular area should be given respect, flexibility, and leadership experiences in the coordination of their programs. Therefore, each program of study (e.g., teacher preparation, exercise science, sports management, health studies) has its own program director or coordinator and a group of faculty with a similar interest. Each director meets with faculty who teach in this area and coordinates course offerings, faculty appointments, and budgets (often in consultation with the department chair or dean, depending on the structure of the unit). The role of the unit manager (chair or dean) is to facilitate the academic programs and coordinators, as well as to keep up with the "dirty work," file-keeping, data analysis, enrollment trends, publicity, facilities management, equipment purchase, and budget preparation.

While faculty work in teams within a particular program area, their interests expand beyond their immediate scholarly areas. It is one thing to promote a certain direction and philosophy, but it is also essential that the program leader become a role model who provides encouragement and support. One overriding perspective, however, is that while each program has some autonomy and flexibility, the faculty are all part of the same department, and must therefore share information and work together. Cross-disciplinary work is critical not only to the program, but also to the future of the profession. It is important that faculty understand and embrace the connections between the subdisciplines. For example, coaches will need to integrate pedagogy, sport sociology, sport psychology, and sports medicine. Likewise, physical educators must combine pedagogy, fitness education, psychology, and exercise physiology in order to teach fitness units, and incorporate philosophy and sport sociology into games and activities in order to promote value education.

Faculty who share information, work together, join committees, participate in interdisciplinary studies, and have experience in research, community service, and university relations do not come about easily. Nor is it easy for a department to develop a reputation as one of the most productive on campus, both in terms of scholarship and service. Below are some of the principles and techniques that can be used to foster these positive characteristics.

In a paper presented on administrative models at the NAPEHE national convention, Seagrave (1993) described the "Feingold Model." He noted that this model "is predicated on the principles of integration and collaboration, the ultimate goal being a professional unification consummated by the marriage of the academic and the practical—the creation of 'a true community of scholars'" (Lidstone & Feingold, 1991, p. 42). He also asserted that "the Feingold Model exhorts both academicians and practitioners to undertake common ventures in efforts to transform social reality, ventures that focus on important social issues." As Rees, Feingold, and Barrette (1991b) reported, "practitioners and academics are beginning to

Administrative Philosophy

Administrative Styles and Models

realize that without each other they cannot successfully set or solve problems" (p. 322). They identified subdisciplinary fragmentation, elitism, and negative stereotyping as impediments to the process of collaboration.

This model tends to follow Boyer's (1990) expanded notion of scholarship, which was further discussed in Fiorentino's (1997) and Feingold's (1997) papers on "service-based scholarship" in *Quest*. If the administration, faculty, and tenure and promotion committee view scholarship in the traditional and narrow role, projects involving community service become difficult to support; hence the importance of laying the groundwork through faculty leadership, collaboration, and networking within the university. It is not unrealistic to expect that committed faculty and strong leadership can help to change or expand traditional views of scholarship to include a more practical or service-related perspective, not only within the unit, but throughout the university. In addition, and most importantly, the model tends to exemplify Sherif's "Super-Ordinate Goal Theory," or shared ownership.

Super-Ordinate Goal Theory

Super-ordinate goals—first identified by social psychologist Sherif (1958) in his study of the interaction between 11-and-12-year-old boys in a summer camp—are those that cannot be achieved without cooperation between potentially competing groups or individuals. In his classic study, Sherif and colleagues observed as animosity increased between two groups of boys, and then tried to find ways to reduce this friction. While it is worth noting that competitive sport provided the context for the development of this conflict, the principal finding of the study was that common goals developed by these competing groups did not decrease the tension. Only when the experimenters introduced superordinate goals—in which the two groups had to coordinate their actions to attain success—was the tension reduced.

Although I was unaware of this theory of "shared ownership" when I began as an administrator, some of my successes as an administrator and leader were the result of following the same principles. The superordinate goal theory is especially valuable when one is trying to get people to work together on joint projects, share information across disciplines, and show more committed effort on projects because of their joint ownership. The principle has worked well, regardless of the population involved (e.g., faculty, youth-sports coaches, medical personnel, social workers, business personnel). It may take a little longer, but the follow-up and commitment benefits are greater. A few of the projects and initiatives that involved working with others (community, schools, higher education) helped to establish a respect for faculty across subdisciplines, thereby developing increased communication and collaboration within the unit.

Little League Project

Application of this theory occurs when individuals and groups work together on a project that will help others. The first such project for our department was a Little League coaches' workshop, one that we have continued to hold for the past 20 years. Faculty in sport sociology, pedagogy, exercise science, motor development, sports medicine, and coaching had to reflect on the most important concepts within their areas of expertise and make them simple enough for laymen to understand. The key to the workshop was that all faculty had to attend each individual's presentation and interject their area of expertise where appropriate. For example, a study on the heart rates of Little League batters showed that the average was 168 bpm, obviously representing high stress. Therefore, one discussion dealt with why children are under this stress and how to reduce it. Also essential to the process was the fact that a group of Little League coaches and leaders met with the faculty on what they thought they needed from the workshop. The workshops have been so successful that the league was written up in *Sports Illustrated* several years ago (Hilgers, 1988) as a model program in which coaches care about their players. The program represents 30 divisions and about 1,000 coaches and 20,000 children in a blue-collar section of Queens.

The significance of that initial workshop was that faculty from all of the subdisciplines within the department worked on the project, heard what each other had to offer, and started a communication network that was invaluable for the development of future projects, especially those that cut across disciplines. Too often, faculty tend to work in isolation, communicate only with those with their same expertise, or develop a hierarchy of the importance of each subdiscipline. For a detailed description of the workshop, see Rees, Feingold, and Barrette (1991a).

The teacher-development team in our unit redesigned our teacher-preparation methods courses to better meet the New York State Standards. This revision began five years after a group of teachers and I had written the standards (called the "Compact for Learning") for New York State in 1989 as a way to convince the state education department that health and physical education deserved to continue as requirements, since they met the state's educational goals. At the time, this represented a significant change of direction for physical education, from focusing only on motor-skill development to promoting lifelong activities, disease prevention, and enhanced personal living skills. In each standard, the focus was on the process, not the product. As these documents filtered through the school districts, physical educators realized that things were changing, and that they did not know how to teach according to the new standards and directions. They came to our department for help, partly because I had written the document, but more so because the department had previously made connections with them and their administrators over the years. Seven of the faculty agreed to hold a workshop for over 90 school districts on Long Island. As a result, the faculty met often and had to immerse themselves in the documents and philosophy. While the two-day workshops were successful (many of the elementary-, middle-, and high-school personnel did indeed change their programs), the faculty concluded that this new direction for schools indicated that they must prepare teachers differently. Because they were all immersed in the new philosophy, it was relatively easy for them to look at each preparatory course and change it, infusing concepts of fitness, personal living skills, and disabilities. Studies by Kowalski (1994), Kowalski and Rizzo (1996), and Fiorentino (1994) showed that these changes have made a difference in our students; since they know how to implement the state standards, they are highly sought after for jobs.

Given our commitment to the schools and our faculty's involvement with the schools through the implementation of the new standards, our department started an advisory committee with school personnel. We realized that public schools and higher education need each other. Too often, university faculty and school teachers criticize each other as being bad

[margin note: Teacher-Preparation Program]

[margin note: Support HPE]

teacher educators or bad teachers. We provide workshops for practitioners, and they provide expertise and valuable experiences for our students. Part of their role on the advisory board is to provide us with information on how we can better prepare our students. Thus we come together as equal partners in the preparation of our future teachers. Our most recent projects include a dual HPE program, a combined exercise-science and pedagogy certificate, and various technology initiatives. For a more detailed description of this support network, see Fiorentino, Kowalski, and Barrette (1993).

Institute for Sports Medicine and Fitness

While superordinate goal theory is an important principle of administration that has played a significant role in our departmental changes, I do not think that it would have had as powerful an impact on us without the development of our Institute for Sports Medicine and Fitness. This institute was created in 1976 for the purpose of developing programs in the community with a clinical component. The Institute allows for creative programming, community-based programs, and special workshops, and it houses our continuing-education programs, coaching certifications, adult-fitness and cardiac-rehabilitation programs, American College of Sports Medicine (ACSM) workshops, and children's swim program. It is our primary outreach endeavor. The adult-fitness program brings the community into the university and at the same time provides experience for our exercise-science students. The ACSM workshops bring in professionals from throughout the east and link the department to valuable hospital personnel and in-service training. The in-service workshops enhance the skills of teachers, coaches, and students. The swim programs bring children to campus—both beginners and competitive swimmers—and again provide valuable experience for our students. Our most recent outreach has been the support of a new program called "Athletes Helping Athletes, Inc." This program provides leadership training for high school athletes on issues such as alcohol, drug abuse, and violence. These athletes, who are hand-picked by their school counselors and athletic directors, then work with middle school students on these issues. Since many are role models in their respective schools, it is anticipated that they will have a positive impact on younger children. Again, I have brought our social-science team in to evaluate the effectiveness of the program. We have also brought our own students in to help with these leadership workshops; when they intern in the schools, they become assistants for the program. Without the Institute, I would never have been able to obtain funding for programs like this. The funding comes from the money brought into the Institute as a result of its various workshops, training courses, and educational programs.

The ultimate value of the Institute is its ability to open up funding and support lines for faculty and equipment and to hire full-time staff in cardiac rehabilitation, adult fitness, and aquatics. The incentives discussed previously can be brought to fruition through the Institute, and it buys a great deal of freedom for the chair. If someone has a good idea, we can get support for it. The Institute is a win-win concept. It brings in the community, provides support for those who wish to cultivate an idea, provides valuable clinical experiences for students, and makes money for the university.

Summary

Leading faculty through the changing higher-education matrix requires an administrator who is a role model—one who participates in all areas of the university, has a passion for the profession, and is willing to reach out to the community. Bringing faculty together with other groups for problem-solving or project development enables faculty to network and establish future collaboration on critical projects. Through this networking and collaboration, faculty can expand their vision and expertise and, in so doing, increase their scholarly inquiry, curricular development, and teaching skills, all of which will enhance the reputation of the unit. The credibility of a unit and its faculty will endure through a variety of educational changes. It is a lot better to be a leader in times of change than to follow.

About the Author

Ronald S. Feingold has been chair of the Department of Physical Education and Human Performance Science at Adelphi University in New York for 27 years. Eight years ago, the health-studies department was placed under his responsibility, and the department's name was changed to Health Studies, Physical Education, and Human Performance Science. Professor Feingold is a past president of AAHPERD, EDA, NYSAHPERD, and NAPEHE, and is current president of AIESEP (International Association for Physical Education in Higher Education). He has also been chairman of the board for the Long Island chapter of the American Heart Association, and president of the university's faculty senate on three separate occasions.

References

Boyer, E. (1990). *Scholarship reconsidered: Priorities of the professorate.* Princeton, NJ: The Carnegie Foundation.

Feingold, R. S. (1997). Service-based scholarship. *Quest, 49*(4), 351-354.

Fiorentino, L. (1994, June). *Dimensions of programmatic effects: Qualitative analysis of student perceptions.* Paper presented at AIESEP World Congress, Berlin.

Fiorentino, L. (1997). Service-based scholarship: An impetus for change in higher education. *Quest, 49*(4), 369-379.

Fiorentino, L., Kowalski, E., & Barrette, G. (1993). Support PE: Moving towards collaboration in teacher preparation. *The Journal of Physical Education, Recreation & Dance, 64*(5), 76-83.

Hilgers, L. (1988, August 22). Stress-free Little League. *Sports Illustrated,* 92-93.

Kowalski, E. (1994, June). *A comparative analysis of preservice students' attitudes towards teaching individuals with disabilities.* Paper presented at AIESEP World Congress, Berlin.

Kowalski, E., & Rizzo, T. (1996). Factors influencing preservice student attitudes towards individuals with disabilities. *Adapted Physical Education Quarterly, 13*(2), 180-196.

Lidstone, J., & Feingold, R. S. (1991). Introduction—The case for integration and collaboration. *Quest, 43,* 241-246.

Rees, C. R., Feingold, R. S., & Barrette, G. T. (1991a). Benefiting youth sport—College faculty and volunteer coaches working together equally. *The Journal of Physical Education, Recreation & Dance, 62*(1), 27-31.

Rees, C. R., Feingold, R. S., & Barrette, G. T. (1991b). Overcoming obstacles to collaboration and integration. *Quest, 43*(3), 319-333.

Seagrave, J. (1993). *Chaos in the profession: Past, present, and future alternatives.* Paper presented at the National Association for Physical Education in Higher Education Convention, Ft. Lauderdale, FL.

Sherif, M. (1958). Super-ordinate goals in the reduction of intergroup conflict. *American Journal of Sociology, 63,* 349-356.

9 Communicating with Faculty, Staff, and Students

James E. Bryant, *Professor and Chair Emeritus, San Jose State University*

Personnel management is the most important aspect of a department chair's responsibilities. You are expected to fulfill promises made by your predecesor. Some will suspect you of giving advantage to faculty appointed during your term.

        Marlene Mawson

Effective communication is critical to survival for chairs and deans within health, kinesiology, and leisure-studies (HKLS) units or any other academic discipline. Regardless of your administrative style, if you don't take the time to communicate, you will ultimately position yourself for failure. Chairs and deans have a responsibility to communicate with faculty, staff, and students on a regular basis, in addition to communicating with each other. Deans must also communicate with upper administration through a chain of command beginning with the provost.

In general, communication includes several identifiable components: (1) the source (sender), (2) the message, (3) the channel by which the message is delivered (format), and (4) the receiver (Parks, Zanger, & Quarterman, 1998). Every sender and receiver of a communication attaches meaning to the communicated message. Senders think they know precisely what they are conveying within their messages. However, receivers read body language, look for hidden meanings, and analyze purpose. The perceptions they form become a real part of this communication process, and chairs and deans usually learn early on that they are perceived differently than their academic colleagues. Serving in these administrative roles requires being careful of what you say and how you say it. If you tell a joke that is construed as offensive by just one person, you will be labeled as insensitive. If you make a grammatical error—particularly if you work within a HKLS unit—you may well be identified by some as being limited in your communication skills and, consequently, incapable of leading. Chairs and deans are placed on a pedestal that requires them to perform differently than others within the administrative structure. It is critical that you communicate openly through the use of a variety of different formats. This will give you the opportunity to establish effective dialogue and develop a positive perception of what you are saying and doing.

"Management by Walking" as a Communication Format

"Management by walking" is time-consuming, but from the standpoint of personal interaction it is perhaps the most effective form of communication. When an administrator literally walks among faculty, staff, and students and interacts with them on an informal basis, good things typically result. If you have never "managed by walking," this form of communication may be intimidating to you, depending on your personality and what you want your working relationship to be like. If you are introverted, you will have to force yourself to get out of your office, at least initially. For the extrovert, it's a piece of cake. Regardless of how easy or difficult it is for you to "walk and talk," keep in mind that the goal is to communicate, build trust, and establish a positive working relationship.

Walking and talking with faculty. Faculty tend to be quite territorial. They spend a major portion of their day in the gymnasium, classroom, laboratory, or their office. Their office may well have a carpet on the floor, pictures on the wall, a portable refrigerator snuggled next to their desk, and a radio or CD player; this is their home away from home. Classrooms and labs are similarly personalized. In comparison, your office is considered a sacred place by faculty, even though it may have many of the same comfort items. Your office represents power and authority to them. It is usually located within the main office and protected by staff who question faculty on why they need to see you. There is often a conference room situated adjacent to your office that conveys the same message. Anytime you can disarm faculty and their perception of power and authority by positioning yourself in an informal setting or by addressing them within their own territory, you have situated yourself positively.

You "manage by walking" by doing just that: arm yourself with a notebook, palm pilot, or tape recorder so that you can keep notes of those things you need to remember, and then march down the hallway of your building. Stick your head in the door of a faculty member's office and say hello. Ask how things are going. If you have an agenda or are in need of a sounding board for a particular issue, here is your chance to bring it up. If you want to make it a social call, that is acceptable as well, since a casual conversation opens possible discussion items. You should also stick your head into other settings (e.g., an exercise-physiology lab, an activity class, a coach's office, a sport-management classroom) simply to acknowledge a colleague's existence. Just take care not to interrupt the function of the class or the business within an office.

If you are new in your administrative role or have never managed by walking before, then you are at risk; the reality is that faculty are suspicious of "odd" behavior. If your behavior is out of the ordinary, faculty will be concerned about your motives and agenda. Thus, you will have to "make the walk" on a consistent basis. If you are a chair, do it at least two to three times per week, scattered across various time periods of the day. If you are a dean, you have triple or quadruple the number of faculty to touch base with and less time to do it. When you go to a meeting in the president's office, however, you can walk through the kinesiology department and stick your head into a few offices. Or, when you are on your way to your car for a meeting with city officials, you can go out of your way to walk through the health department. You never know what piece of advice or insight you might receive during these chance contacts.

Keep in mind that if you don't "walk about" on a consistent basis, you will be limited in what you know about your administrative unit, and you will not have the opportunity to share with faculty in an informal manner. As a result, barriers to communication will continue to exist, and your job in the long run will be more difficult.

Walking and talking with staff. Staff members are your professional friends—don't ever forget it! They deserve your loyalty and support whenever possible. After all, it is they who really run the administrative unit. If you are going to succeed in your role, you must communicate with staff through "management by walking."

Staff have the same territorial tendencies as faculty. Your secretaries are limited to the space on their desk, but that's their territory. Your technicians, equipment managers, locker-room attendants, and lab support personnel may have an office or, at the very least, a large work area: that is their territory.

Chairs know where their staff are, and in most cases they have access to them. It is easy to make casual trips by their work areas to discuss issues that are important to them and provide them with insight on what is happening in the department. Secretaries are easier to make contact with because of their location in your work vicinity, but don't be misled into thinking that you are automatically in touch with them. You should avoid the intercom or telephone on occasion in favor of walking up to a secretary's desk and talking. One of the great benefits of doing this is that it familiarizes you with what is really going on in the office (e.g., what problems are the staff experiencing? What bothers them, and what makes them feel good?). Be prepared to engage in dialogue that is meaningful, and don't forget to listen. If you are a dean, the same advice applies with your immediate staff; remember that your staff is also composed of those workers within all the departments in your unit. Be sure to walk about and see staff in each of the departments. Get to know them on a first-name basis and discuss issues that are important to them.

Walking and talking with students. Student territory is limited. Undergraduate students don't have an office, a work area, or a desk that they can call their own. Graduate students sometimes have a territory, usually limited to a carrel, a desk, or in some cases an office. If you took a poll concerning your identity and role as a chair, you would find that most undergraduates don't have a clue about who you are or what you do. Graduate students may know who you are if you have engaged them in a personal interview before appointing them to assistantships, but others may not know you at all. If you are a dean, it is pretty much guaranteed that a poll would reveal that neither the undergraduate nor the graduate students even know your name, let alone what you do.

These facts alone are a good enough reason to stop and talk to students on occasion. Look for groups of them and insert yourself into their conversation. Ask questions, listen, and engage in casual conversation. Drop by a recreation-therapy classroom or stress-management lab before class and joke with them, or go by the graduate students' "office area" and socialize for a few minutes, just as you do with faculty. Initially, you may have to introduce yourself, but if you make it a habit to talk to students, they will learn who you are and welcome your intrusions.

Written Forms of Communication

Various types of written communication are available and should be used to communicate with faculty, staff, and students. Again, the way you use these communication tools may be different depending on whether you are a chair or dean. Furthermore, these tools should be used in combination with each other for maximum effectiveness.

Memos. Memos are best used for formal communication. They are used as cover letters for a hard copy of statistical or factual information and to put formal opinions or statements in writing.

Memos are often used in personnel situations. If a faculty or staff member needs to be reprimanded, the reprimand typically comes in the form of a memo (figure 9.1). On the other hand, a compliment or congratulatory message is also appropriate through a memo.

Writing a memo to summarize an understanding of the content of a meeting (figure 9.2) is often a valuable form of communication, particularly when misrepresentation has occurred after previous meetings. Vision statements or summaries at the beginning or end of a semester or academic year are also appropriate occasions for memos (figure 9.3). These types of memos give faculty and staff a focus for a projected period of time, or issues for reflection. They also document administrative intent.

Good advice regarding memos is, "Don't put anything in writing that you are not willing to back up," and, "Don't write a memo when a spoken comment will have more of an impact." The bottom line is that a memo is a formal means of communication that is designed to be used selectively.

FIGURE 9.1
Reprimand

Memo

January 24, 2001

To: Jonathon Smith, Associate Professor, Leisure Studies
From: Jane Brown, Chair, Leisure Studies
Re: Faculty Meeting Attendance

This is to remind you of university policy regarding mandatory attendance at department faculty meetings. Per our conversation of January 23, 2001, you are reminded that university policy requires that attendance at formal planned faculty meetings is mandatory, and absence from a meeting requires prior approval of the chair. Please see Faculty Handbook Sect. 4.1, "Faculty Meeting Attendance."

If you are absent without prior approval again, I am required by policy to file a formal statement for your Personnel Action File, and subsequent absences without approval will result in docking of your pay.

FIGURE 9.2
Understanding of
Content

Memo

January 24, 2001

To: Mary Creek, Associate Faculty Affairs Director
From: Jason Horn, Dean, Health and Human Performance
Re: Summary of Meeting of January 23, 2001

Mary, this is a brief summary of what I understood from our conversation regarding the university grievance procedure and faculty tenure responses.

As outlined by you on January 23, 2001, I understand that my responsibility regarding the recent grievance filed by Dr. Jerri Oates, Professor of Kinesiology, is to....

Would you please confirm that my understanding is consistent with our conversation, and that this is the way we plan on proceeding in reference to the....

FIGURE 9.3
Focus

Memo

August 24, 2000

To: Colleagues
From: Bill Jorgenson, Dean, Kinesiology and Health Science
Re: Academic Year 2000-01

Our new academic year 2000-01 holds great promise for a productive and successful year. From a resource standpoint, we have received an increase of 8 percent in our state allocation budget, and our fundraising efforts have generated a marked increase of 24 percent. We have also....

As a result of increased resources, support from the office of the provost on strategic planning, and the increase of 18 percent in the number of majors across the departmental units, we have the potential to make significant progress with three major goals for the new academic year. The first of these goals....

Voice mail is designed for brief messages directed to individuals or groups. Use of voice mail should be limited to informational items or requests that require quick responses. One irritation for faculty is to have to listen to multiple and lengthy messages, whether they are relevant or not. Plan what you are going to say in advance so that you can be specific, short, and direct; this will be appreciated far more than a long-winded and general discussion of a topic.

E-mail. We live in a electronic age that requires us to take advantage of technology to enhance our ability to communicate. It is important to understand, however, that not all faculty are excited about such technology. The use of e-mail can be a threat to their traditional ways of doing things. Dealing with this given is important, but at the same time, it is necessary to establish an intra-departmental communication format dependent, to some degree, on technology.

A couple of suggestions may make life easier for you. First, if you are a chair, establish or expand an intra-departmental listserv for faculty, graduate assistants, staff, and students. You can build this system in a variety of ways. For example, you could establish one listserv for faculty and staff, a second that includes everyone except students, and a third that is for students only. If you are a dean, you are probably restricted to two listserv audiences: one each for the chairs and faculty in your school or college.

Faculty and staff who really don't want to be bothered may create a small glitch in moving forward with a listserv. There is a simple, relatively painless solution to this problem, though: establish a deadline for people to sign on to the listserv (see table 9.1). You will receive criticism from some faculty while being lauded by others. You can involve faculty in the setting of these deadlines, but be sure to set them and move on; in the long run, it will work out. You should not use such deadlines with student listserv users.

A listserv offers a tremendous number of possibilities for communication. Agendas and minutes of meetings can be conveyed, and information and ideas can be shared. The e-mail medium is prone to excessive input, however. Take care not to waste faculty, staff, or student time with inane or wordy messages; communicate in a succinct and direct manner.

TABLE 9.1
Timeline
for Listserv Operation

What to Do	Length of Time
Allow time for personnel to sign on to the listserv	Eight weeks
Provide a viable in-service experience	Early within the eight-week period
Hold to the initial deadline for beginning the listserv	Last day of the eight weeks
For those who are not signed on, copy e-mail messages and post them for faculty to read	For four weeks after listserv begins operation
End copying and posting of e-mail messages	After a total of 12 weeks

It is important to remember that people do not necessarily read their e-mail every day; consequently, it is not the best medium for an urgent message requiring a quick response. If you expect a timely response, you may need to establish some sort of protocol for a return message. A three-working-day minimum for a response is probably a reasonable one, with a week serving as the maximum time expectation. If you allow longer than a week, the message will likely be forgotten, and less than three days may not give faculty enough time to receive and digest the message. Chairs and deans can reasonably request that faculty access their e-mail at home, particularly during summers and between sessions. Most university decisions seem timed for action when everyone except for upper administration is off campus. These items require a quick turnaround, and if you are inclined to involve others in decision-making, there needs to be a communication format that allows you to reach many people quickly.

Newsletters. Newsletters provide a unique form of communication. They are designed for a more long-range effect than other types of communication, and may be delivered in either print or electronic format. A weekly or biweekly newsletter for faculty allows a chair to provide informational material, thought pieces, and an update on the progress of projects and programs. A dean can produce a similar newsletter, but should do it on a monthly rather than weekly basis. Samples of content for a faculty/staff newsletter are listed in table 9.2

If you are a chair, publication of a monthly newsletter for students can be very important. In fact, it may be your main way to communicate with students. The content of such a newsletter will vary, but some examples are presented in table 9.3. You should give the newsletter a name (e.g., *The Communicator; Student Alert; Student Chronicle*).

As a chair or dean, you have to meet with faculty, staff, and students on a formal basis. Meetings can be classified as a major form of communication, and how well-prepared you are will have a lot to do with whether or not you can successfully communicate with your various constituencies.

Interactive Forms of Communication

Faculty and chair meetings. Some faculty just love meetings, while others most certainly do not. Either way, when you hold a meeting with faculty, you must have a purpose, be extremely well-prepared, and systematically structure the proceedings. You will need to hold such meetings on a regular basis (e.g., every two weeks or once per month).

Deans are constantly going to one sort of meeting or another, so planning a chair's meeting on a regular basis may not be a high priority for them. If a dean takes that attitude, however, then disaster is on the horizon. A dean has to make special preparation for a chair's meeting. Chairs need to feel that they have input into the dean's decision-making. Deans also have a responsibility to conduct meetings with unit faculty. This is particularly true at the beginning of a semester, since that is when the tone is set for the entire session. It is important to involve faculty from the various disciplines within the school or college in the planning process. Prepare an interesting "State of the School/College Address," and provide a means for dialogue to occur with faculty. If you can accomplish this, then you are well on your way to being a successful communicator.

TABLE 9.2
Faculty/Staff
Newsletter Content

Title	Content
Communique from the chair or dean	A sharing of information or insight regarding higher-education issues related to the unit
Calendar dates	A list of calendar dates related to the HKLS unit
University or school/college issues	A discussion section reflecting specific issues that might impact the HKLS unit
Advising information	An example of a special section to assist faculty with their responsibilities
Faculty senate information	A summary of faculty senate actions that are critical to the HKLS unit; written by the faculty representative
Staff reminders	A sharing of due dates or reminders for faculty (e.g., regarding how to use the new copier)
In-service section	A column on higher-education learning experiences (e.g., a section on computers or teaching hints)

Staff meetings. Staff are often neglected when it comes to group meetings. As a chair, you should plan at least one staff meeting per semester, depending on the size of your department. In addition, you should meet with your secretarial staff, your locker-room attendants, and your lab technicians on a weekly basis for at least 30 minutes. Monday mornings serve as a logical and appropriate time for such meetings. If your staff is large enough to have supervisors in these areas, then you don't need to hold weekly meetings with all staff in these positions; instead, meet with the supervisors. These meetings are designed to maintain a reciprocal flow of information. Staff can make your job easier if you show them respect by listening to them, meeting with them, and following up their suggestions with action.

Again, if you are a dean, you not only have a staff of your own to deal with, but also the staff of each department within your unit. You should meet with your own staff each Monday. Then, at least once a semester, you should meet with every staff member in the unit collectively. You should also consider having your administrative assistant represent you by meeting with unit staff on a monthly basis.

TABLE 9.3
Student Newsletter
Content

Title	Content
Chair's message	Provide information for students or a thought piece that challenges them to think and discuss
Department/university	A list of dates for drop/add, application for graduation, etc., deadlines
Professional conference dates	List conferences and dates (e.g., AAHPERD National Convention and Exposition, state and district AAHPERD conferences, speciality organization conferences)
Major club	A club representative or sponsor can give you material regarding club activities
Student-leader feature	Feature a student each month
Faculty/staff profile	Feature a faculty or staff member each month
Department news	Share information on new faculty appointments, dates for interviews of candidates for a faculty position, curriculum changes, etc.

Meet with students. Meeting with students is imperative. In some institutions, chairs and deans have been successful in hosting "Coffee with the Dean" or "Have a Pepsi with the Chair" meetings with small groups. Another successful strategy is to organize a monthly meeting with student leaders from the department's major club and speak for 10 minutes on what is current in the unit. In addition, you can open communication lines by sponsoring a "Meet the Chair" or "Meet the Dean" format similar to the TV show, *Meet the Press.* You can use this forum to answer questions, pose some of your own, and generate the view that you are approachable.

On an informal basis, some often overlooked ways of meeting with students include playing in a student-faculty softball game, being a subject during a "Health, Stress, and Fitness Test Day," or serving as a resource person during a "Leisure Career Day." Meetings can also be reduced in size. Whether you are a chair or dean, you should also reserve an "open door" time for students to meet with you (to bring grievances or to simply share with you).

Summary

Communication is critical to your success as a chair or dean within HKLS. Take advantage of the opportunities that open communication affords and the relationships that you establish as a result of such communication. As a chair, take the opportunity to involve the dean in communication within your department. As a dean, use proven communication techniques to advance the role of the unit and assist those who function within it. Remember—the more you communicate, the more you learn. The more you learn, the more effective you can be at enriching the educational experiences of students and assisting faculty in their growth and development.

About the Author

James E. Bryant is a professor and chair emeritus at San Jose State University. He has accumulated 14 years of experience as a chair, and he is a former NAPEHE president and a recipient of the College and University Administrators Council Honor Award.

References

Parks, J. B., Zanger, B. R. K., & Quarterman, J. (1998). *Contemporary sport management*. Champaign, IL: Human Kinetics.

10 Leadership Behavior and Conflict Management

Charles W. Ash, *Chair and Professor, Department of Health, Physical Education, and Sport Science, Kennesaw State University*

John D. Massengale, *Professor, Department of Kinesiology, University of Nevada–Las Vegas*

Pause before making a decision. Sit on it. Give serious thought.

⊶ Charles W. Ash

This chapter contains information and suggestions from the leadership-behavior and conflict-management literature that might best be described as practical administrative remedies for health, physical education, recreation, and dance (HPERD) units. Leadership behavior will be emphasized, with a focus on how leaders can avoid creating a work environment wherein difficult people negatively influence the group. It should be noted that the information presented here is of a very positive nature, emphasizing that cohesion is the best method of leading individuals (however difficult they may be), since it removes the source of many types of conflict.

Leadership Behavior

Leadership behavior is one of the least understood social phenomena in modern society (Burns, 1978). The late Ralph M. Stogdill, who is often recognized as America's greatest contributor to the leadership-behavior literature, suggested that there are almost as many definitions of leadership as there are people who have tried to define it (Bass, 1990). When modern definitions of leadership are examined, many different words and concepts emerge, such as group process, personality, behavior, power, relationship, goals, influence, and persuasion. Northouse (1997) offered a simple and popular definition: "Leadership is a process whereby an individual influences a group of individuals to achieve a common goal" (p. 3). Sometimes, leadership behavior is described in a light-hearted manner, as in a quote attributed to former President Harry Truman: "A leader is a person who has the ability to get other people to do what they don't want to do and like it" (Murray & Mann, 1998). For the purposes of this chapter, the authors would like to offer the following definition: *Leadership is getting people to do what needs to done.* While you are "getting people to do

97

what needs to be done," one factor must remain of primary importance: *professional integrity.* This is an indispensable part of effective leadership behavior, as is well documented in numerous studies reported in the literature (Bass, 1990).

How Effective Leaders Act

Leaders do make a difference. According to Tucker (1981), there is always an act of leadership in the beginning; there is no such thing as a leaderless movement. Leadership is always situational, however (Fiedler, 1967). Being an effective leader in one situation does not automatically mean that a person will be an effective leader in an entirely different situation. For instance, the recognized leader of a motorcycle gang may be an effective leader, but in all probability would fail as a military officer or the head of a church.

With this in mind, and considering some of the most current and extensive leadership-behavior literature available (Bass, 1990; Bogue, 1985; Cangemi, Kowalski, & Khan, 1998; Northouse, 1997), a pattern of effective leadership behavior can be established with certainty.

- *Effective leadership behavior is always related to social power, exchange, and influence.* Good leaders have good social skills. Personality differences may be more or less well received in certain situations.
- *Good leaders have the ability to create and maintain groups.* Group maintenance often becomes a leader's top priority, since it is best achieved through successful performance.
- *Excellent leaders are always intelligent.* Plainly stated, there are no dumb leaders. Regardless of situations and perceptions, people with only average intelligence have little chance of becoming successful leaders.
- *Leaders tend to be dominant, assertive, and self-confident; they seek responsibility and authority, and generally have higher levels of aspiration.* Leaders are very optimistic; they are usually confident that they can do something, and often succeed.
- *It is hard to find effective leaders who do not have high levels of technical competency.* Leaders are good at whatever they are leading in.
- *Strong leaders always display high levels of enthusiasm.* Enthusiasm is contagious in a group situation. There are no unenthusiastic leaders. They may have dramatically different personalities or be in very different situations, but they will somehow display passion and enthusiasm.
- *People who establish themselves as effective leaders always have a tremendous capacity for hard work.* They often demonstrate their leadership behavior by working past normal working hours.
- *Effective leaders develop the ability to use minimal verbiage while at the same time developing excellent communication skills.* High-level communication skills always accompany high-level leadership skills.
- *Finally, the most recent literature reveals the importance of a sense of humor.* Although it may be demonstrated in many different ways, good leaders always have a good sense of humor.

How Leaders Make Groups More Cohesive

One of the best methods of dealing with difficult people and reducing potential conflict is to take positive and assertive action toward making a group more cohesive. There are a number of ways to do this, and what follow are suggestions that were specifically selected for individuals with strong backgrounds in sport and physical activity, such as those typically found in academic units of HPERD.

First and foremost, the group must become a bona fide group, not merely a collection of people. This process is absolutely necessary; otherwise, any attempt at strong leadership behavior will be met by resistance, conflict, and disarray. Carron (1994) suggested that cohesion in a group can be accomplished through the following: the development of a strong collective identity; a shared purpose; highly structured patterns of interaction and communication; clearly defined personal and task interdependence, with accompanying role acceptance and responsibility; and a strong sense of personal attraction.

One effective group-building technique for people with strong sport and physical activity backgrounds can be found in the principle of *proximity*. When people are physically close to one another, bonding tends to occur. This principle has been examined for years and can be seen in athletic dorms, locker rooms, and training-table meals, in the territorialism related to facilities and equipment, and even in the clustering of offices in a HPERD unit. Proximity can build stronger groups that become capable of real cohesiveness.

Norms should also be established. Common standards of behavior for a group are strongly associated with cohesion. When a group accepts norms, the result is often conformity in expected behavior, which limits the power of difficult people and lessens the opportunity for conflict. The creation and support of norms is an important part of good leadership behavior.

Another group-building technique involves the principle of *similarity*. The more similar the members of a group, the more likely they will remain compatible, thereby causing fewer conflicts for one another. Diversity has become an expectation in contemporary higher education, but within diversity there still remains the opportunity to discover similarities (i.e., where people are more alike than different). Highlighting these similarities leads to group cohesion and fewer opportunities for conflict.

Strong *commitment* is also common to the members and leaders of cohesive groups. True commitment is clearly visible; it requires personal sacrifice from everyone in the group, functioning as a bonding agent and leading to personal and group satisfaction.

Last, but not least, is the importance of *distinctiveness*. The more a group distances and distinguishes itself from others, the more the group members develop a feeling of unity. That feeling leads directly to cohesion. Members of HPERD units in the U.S. are, in most cases, products of the American educational and athletic system. They eagerly respond to—and believe in—that which makes them distinctive. In most cases, they like uniforms, logos, mottoes, rites of passage, and the special privileges that accompany initiation. Distinctiveness is considered by many to be even more powerful than proximity. Whether it's the haircut of a U.S Marine, the plain black football jersey of an Oakland Raider, or the unique letterhead of a college of health and human performance, it works.

Even with all of these techniques of good leadership, how do you deal with conflict? As in other academic disciplines, conflicts are a given within an HPERD unit. The issue for administrators is how to help colleagues manage these conflicts before they become disruptive to the unit climate. Conflict can occur between a HPERD chair and faculty as a result of the chair's leadership responsibilities (e.g., annual performance evaluations,

Conflict Management

tenure and promotion recommendations, merit salary awards, travel awards, teaching assignments, summer contracts, committee assignments). Conflicts can also occur between a chair and an upper administrator (e.g., dean or vice president) and between faculty and students. Every administrator has S.O.P.s (Sources of Pain) among the faculty (Bell & Smith, 1997). How you manage these S.O.P.s will determine the level of conflict in your unit.

In a study conducted by the Center for the Study of the Department Chair at the University of Washington (Gmelch & Miskin, 1993), it was found that conflict with colleagues was a major source of stress for department chairs. The primary stressors identified in this study were (1) making decisions affecting others (identified by 45 percent of the respondents), (2) resolving collegial differences (45 percent), (3) evaluating faculty performance (42 percent), (4) resolving differences with superiors (17 percent), and (5) resolving differences with students (5 percent). Dealing with administrative red tape was identified as the most dissatisfying task required of a chair. However, high on the list of dissatisfying tasks were the above duties, as well as dealing with inter-faculty conflict, negative faculty attitudes, and non-supportive faculty.

Resolution of all conflict is the ultimate goal of an HPERD administrator. However, since conflict is inevitable in every unit, "managing" it becomes the more realistic goal. The process of establishing policies regarding inter-personal behaviors in a unit (e.g., "agreeing to disagree" on issues) will ultimately lead unit members to understand what is appropriate and inappropriate behavior, thus leading to more effective conflict management.

Conflict is not always inappropriate. In fact, constructive conflict allows for differences of opinion, as long as they concern issues and not people or personalities. The academy has had as its cornerstone the belief that anyone may advance an idea without fear of reprisals. Growth and advancement is the product of open, honest, philosophical debates. On the other hand, disruptive or personal conflict can have serious repercussions regarding open debate on issues. This type of conflict has a negative effect on the morale and growth of the faculty and climate of the unit.

Leaming (1998) and Lucas (1994) offered the following very important practical strategies for all administrators to use when developing human-relationship and leadership skills and managing dysfunctional conflict between faculty.

Be clear in communicating goals and expectations for the department. All faculty in the unit must understand the policies and procedures of both the unit and the institution. More important, the chair must be consistent in applying these policies to all faculty to avoid conflict and the perception of favoritism. This will protect the chair from potential accusations of arbitrary and capricious treatment in a grievance or litigation.

Establish ground rules with the faculty for handling disagreements and be consistent in adhering to these rules. Establish procedures to follow when conflicts arise. The most universal procedure is if one faculty member has a complaint or concern about another faculty member, then the complainant should discuss the issue with the other faculty member rather than with a third faculty member. If the two faculty members cannot resolve the issue, then the chair may intervene as a mediator. Additionally, the chair can recommend conflict mediation through the institution's office of conflict management. This latter option should always be the course of action if there is a perception by either faculty member that the chair may be biased.

Anticipate and be prepared to intervene in areas where conflict may occur. In many situations, an administrator can usually anticipate when an issue is going to be controversial and potentially lead to conflict. It is in the best interests of the unit if the administrator plans ahead in an attempt to reduce, as much as possible, the impact of the issue.

A good administrator must be a good listener. In many cases, faculty just want someone to listen to them as they vent their frustration. However, when problems surface, it is important to focus your energy into active listening.

Keep an open-door policy. By being visible and providing opportunities for faculty to visit you in your office, you will enhance the positive climate of the department and decrease the likelihood of conflict. Additionally, if you attempt to visit the faculty in their offices or in the hallways, it will add to the perception that you truly care about them as colleagues. You can never do too much LWA (Leadership by Walking Around).

When you make a mistake, admit it. Everyone makes mistakes; it takes a person of integrity to admit it. In the eyes of your colleagues, your value as an administrator will be significantly enhanced if you admit and learn from your mistakes.

Look for ways to compliment faculty members. There is nothing that succeeds like success. When faculty members accomplish something, compliment them among their colleagues in the unit and find ways to promote their accomplishments throughout the institution. The best way to change negative behavior is to accentuate the positive.

Treat everyone honestly and fairly. Be open and honest on issues. Evaluate faculty in relation to departmental and institutional expectations for faculty performance. Assign workloads, merit raises, travel monies, teaching times, and so forth as fairly as possible. It is also wise to publish as much of this information as you can so that perceptions and reality coincide.

Write things down. The number of individuals seen by an administrator in a day or week is often staggering. Coupled with this contact itself is the number of requests that permeate each conversation. Thus it is best to write things down as they come to you so that you have a record of each request or event. Additionally, such notes become reminders to follow-up on an issue. Remember, the amount of time needed to make a decision is directly proportional to the importance of the decision. Try to avoid snap decisions.

Compromising is not necessarily a sign of weakness. Everyone has probably heard the axiom: "Life is a series of compromises." In administration, this is very true. The higher you go in administration, the greater the expectation that you exhibit a global perspective on issues. Make strong cases where they should be made, and don't compromise on your ethical, moral, or professional values. In other words, "choose your battles wisely"!

You are "their" chairperson, but they are not "your" faculty. As a department chair, you are considered "first among your colleagues." You have been placed in a position of leadership, hopefully with the confidence and support of each faculty member in the unit. The success of the unit is not a result of your reign over the faculty, however, but rather of the cooperation and respect exhibited by the faculty in striving for the common goals of the unit. Chairs are sometimes perceived by faculty as being "neither fish nor fowl." That is to say, you have one role as a faculty member ("we") in the unit, but another, perhaps contradictory, role as an administrator ("they"). These "we" versus "they" roles can sometimes lead to conflict.

A faculty member is not necessarily wrong just because she or he sees things and behaves differently than you. I am reminded of a plaque that I saw hanging in a fellow coach's office back in the 1970s that read, "The Coach's Rules: Rule #1—The Coach is always right. Rule #2—See Rule #1." This approach might work in coaching, but seldom does it work when one is attempting to develop a cohesive academic unit. I am also reminded of a popular Southern saying: "There's more than one way to skin a cat." Every issue has many points of view and potential solutions, depending on the perspective of the faculty member involved. The richness of the discussion and the decision-making process is a result of these various points of view.

Summary

The authors of this chapter recommend that aspiring, new, or veteran administrators become familiar with the leadership and conflict-management literature. If your institution has a center for conflict management or provides training in this area, you should take advantage of these opportunities to become better prepared to meet the challenges of leadership and conflict management in your academic unit. Additionally, seek out administrative colleagues on your campus or in professional organizations (e.g., CUAC and NAPEHE) regarding common issues and concerns. As you begin to confide in them and discuss leadership and conflict-management issues, you will quickly realize that most administrators have dealt with these issues and are willing to share their experiences.

Administrators must continue to explore the literature and attend conferences and workshops on leadership and conflict-management issues. These topics, and most of the others found in this book, can be found in the references listed at the end of each chapter. Furthermore, Kansas State University holds a conference every year in Florida on topics specific to the role of the department chair in an academic unit. The American Council on Education conducts three workshops every year in various regions of the country for new deans and chairs. Many colleges and universities (e.g., Kennesaw State University in Georgia) provide workshops for administrators to engage in discussion on many administrative issues. All administrators, whether new or seasoned, should take advantage of these opportunities to enhance their skills in the areas of leadership and conflict management.

About the Authors

Charles W. Ash is a chair and professor in the Department of Health, Physical Education, and Sport Science at Kennesaw State University in Georgia. He has been in higher education for 32 years, with experience in three state systems (Vermont, New York, and Georgia).

John D. Massengale is a professor in the Department of Kinesiology at the University of Nevada, Las Vegas. He has more than 30 years of experience in higher education, with appointments as professor, head football coach, department chair, and dean.

References

Bass, B. M. (1990). *Handbook of leadership*. New York: The Free Press.

Bell, A. H., & Smith, D. M. (1997). *Winning with difficult people.* Hauppauge, NY: Barron's.

Bogue, E. G. (1985). *The enemies of leadership*. Bloomington, IN: Phi Delta Kappa.

Burns, J. M. (1978). *Leadership*. New York: Harper & Row.

Cangemi, J. P., Kowalski, C. J., & Khan, K. H. (1998). *Leadership behavior*. New York: University Press of America.

Carron, A. V. (1994). Group dynamics in sport. In S. Serpa, J. Alves, & V. Pataco (Eds.), *International perspective on sport and exercise psychology* (pp. 79-101). Morgantown, WV: Fitness Information Technology.

Fiedler, F. (1967). *A theory of leadership effectiveness*. New York: McGraw-Hill.

Gmelch, W. H., & Miskin, V. D. (1993). *Leadership skills for department chairs.* Boston: Anker.

Leaming, D. R. (1998). *Academic leadership: A practical guide to chairing the department.* Boston: Anker.

Lucas, A. F. (1994). *Strengthening departmental leadership: A team-building guide for chairs in colleges and universities.* San Francisco: Jossey-Bass.

Murray, M. C., & Mann, B. L. (1998). Leadership effectiveness. In J. M. Williams (Ed.), *Applied sport psychology* (pp. 92-114). Mountain View, CA: Mayfield.

Northouse, P. G. (1997). *Leadership*. Thousand Oaks, CA: Sage.

Tucker, R. C. (1981). *Politics as leadership*. Columbia, MO: University of Missouri Press.

Additional Resources

Fisher, R., & Ury, W. (1991). *Getting to yes: Negotiating agreement without giving in.* New York: Penguin.

Gmelch, W. H., & Miskin, V. D. (1995). *Chairing an academic department.* Thousand Oaks, CA: Sage.

Hecht, I. W. D., Higgerson, M. L., Gmelch, W. H., & Tucker, A. (1999). *The department chair as academic leader.* Phoenix, AZ: Oryx.

Higgerson, M. L. (1996). *Communication skills for department chairs.* Boston: Anker.

Tucker, A. (1993). *Chairing the academic department.* Phoenix, AZ: Oryx.

11 Successfully Conducting Meetings and Retreats

Donna Phillips, *Professor and Chair, Physical Education Department, Western Illinois University*

Become a good listener if you aren't already. Keep confidential your conversations with faculty. Be supportive and positive.

⌗— Donna Phillips

Now that you are initiated as a department chair, it is time to plan your first faculty meeting. The faculty's perceptions of you as the chair of their department will be drastically changed from those that they had of you as a fellow faculty member. As the chair, you are now in the leadership position rather than simply part of the group. One of your important responsibilities in this position is to plan, organize, and conduct faculty meetings and retreats.

Leading faculty meetings is both an art and a science. Good meetings run smoothly and efficiently, are well-planned and organized, adhere to the agenda, and proceed in a timely manner. At the conclusion of a faculty meeting, everyone should leave believing that something positive has been accomplished.

Faculty meetings are an important source of face-to-face communication. Some types of information can be relayed effectively through e-mail or memos, but for important issues and concerns, a meeting is necessary. A meeting should be a forum where new ideas can be freely presented and discussed and where current departmental practices can be examined. Ideally, a successful meeting would culminate with a blend of both old and new ideas and practices.

Scheduling Meetings

Whether you are scheduling a special committee meeting, a regular faculty meeting, or a retreat, scheduling the meeting time is an important factor to consider. If there is a pre-designated time when all faculty are available, the meetings should be scheduled for then. If there is not a designated time, it is your responsibility to find a time when all the faculty are available (i.e., when they have no instructional assignments). It can be difficult to find such a time during the normal daily schedule, so meeting times outside the regular working day may be your best option (e.g., breakfast meetings and meetings after 5:00 p.m.). The pros and cons of each of these times should be considered, and your decision should be based on which time appears to be the most advantageous.

One drawback to meeting outside of the traditional work day is that faculty driving from a distance will have to leave home very early (or get home very late) in order to attend. Further, your support staff may not be available at these times. One advantage of these times, though, is the limited number of outside interferences (e.g., students would not be in the building, the main office would not be open, telephone calls would not be a problem). Thus, the time actually spent in the meeting would be productive. If a meeting is held after 5:00 p.m., you might also discover that faculty are more attentive and the meeting time is more productive because faculty are eager to end their day.

When establishing the starting time of a meeting, consider a time other than on the hour (e.g., 2:35 p.m. or 10:05 a.m.). Strange as it may seem, when you establish such off-hour start times, more people will make it to the meeting on time. This strategy also provides a few free minutes for faculty to interact with one another and engage in conversation that is not directly related to the meeting agenda. In many cases, this interaction is positive and relaxes those in attendance. If you do schedule a meeting on the hour, people will tend to be about five minutes late. You should start the meeting at whatever time you have posted as the beginning time, however. Do not let people get into the habit of arriving 5 to 10 minutes late, believing that you will not begin until they are present.

After you have established a beginning time for a meeting, you should also establish the ending time. You always have the flexibility, with the agreement of those present, to extend the meeting time, but ideally you should adhere to the announced time commitments.

The Meeting Agenda

As you begin the process of planning a scheduled faculty meeting, your first task will be to develop a meeting agenda. Think of the agenda as the blueprint or recipe for a successful meeting.

Before you prepare the agenda, you should ask yourself, "Is this meeting really necessary?" If the answer is yes, then you should determine the purpose(s) of the meeting. If the meeting is not necessary, do not schedule it. Unnecessary meetings are generally unproductive. Once you have determined the purpose(s) of the meeting, your next charge is to develop the agenda. A meeting without an agenda has no focus or direction. Without an agenda, personal issues that are not directly related to the topics being discussed can easily slip into the conversation. Once this happens, the meeting changes from its original purpose into a forum for personal agendas.

It is important to remember that the best meetings occur when new viewpoints or concepts are generated or when policy is developed. Ineffective meetings are those in which the only items on the agenda are individual reports on various projects (Burleson, 1990). Keeping this in mind, you should include discussion time as an agenda item if it is appropriate. If you will be asking for a summary of committee actions, those reports should not be items for discussion, and the summaries should be brief.

Arranging the agenda so that the meeting concludes on a positive note and has the general approval of the faculty is another good strategy. When a meeting is called for a single purpose, it is a good idea to begin the agenda with a statement about this purpose.

An agenda can be long and detailed or short and more topical. Regardless of its form, an agenda presents the flow pattern for discussion items. In its simplest form, an agenda may be a listing of announcements and the order in which items will be discussed. In its more complex forms, a well-planned agenda may serve as a catalyst for developing new policy or practices. An agenda can also serve as a rescue agent to cease discussion on topics that are not directly related to it.

Agendas should be distributed to the attendees at least a week in advance. When possible, agenda items should be phrased more as positive opportunities for discussion than as problems. Most faculty meetings require a multi-topic agenda. The following factors are important when developing such an agenda:

1. List the topics that must be covered. The objective is to limit the meeting to those topics which are essential, timely, and needful of the group's attention.

2. Organize the topics to produce a logical order. Keep related topics together on the agenda so the discussion can flow from one to the next with a minimum of overlap and repeat discussion.

3. With the topics in line, look for evidence of the umbrella syndrome. The umbrella syndrome occurs when agenda items are too generalized, thus leading to discussions that are too broad. To avoid this, each topic should broken into specific agenda items that will facilitate discussion. Moreover, the more specific the topic, the more control you as the leader have over the discussion.

4. When the agenda appears to be complete, survey it for time. If meeting will be too lengthy, divide the agenda into two separate meetings. (The 3-M Meeting Management Team [3M], 1979, pp. 50-51)

Once the agenda has been developed, the next step is to prepare yourself for conducting the meeting. If the meeting is always held in the same room, then you will already be familiar with its layout (e.g., seating arrangements). If the location is not always the same, it is your responsibility to explore possibilities and select a room that best meets the needs of the group. In this age of technological innovation, there are many software presentation programs (e.g., PowerPoint) that can be used during meetings. If you wish to use such tools, you must make arrangements for the set-up of computerized equipment.

Preparation for Conducting a Meeting

Meetings in which the chair is not prepared tend to be ineffective. A visible lack of readiness affects the climate of the entire meeting: "The personality of a meeting is fragile and affected by seemingly small occurrences" (3M, 1979, p. 29). Other factors that contribute to a negative meeting include:

- The chair and/or the participants arriving late.
- The meeting room not being reserved or ready.
- The chair opening the meeting in a jocular manner and encouraging levity.

- The chair appearing unprepared, or opening with a vague statement such as "I'm not sure why I called this meeting but...."
- Participants demonstrating that they aren't ready by fumbling their way through the discussion.
- The meeting being frequently interrupted for telephone or other messages.

The last factor to consider in your meeting preparation is to identify which items on the agenda may be controversial (e.g., a proposal to change the name of the department from "physical education" to "kinesiology"). To do this, you need to: understand how the faculty react to specific issues; know whether the topic has been discussed previously and what the outcome was; and be aware that some faculty will have negotiated prior to the meeting to gain support from other colleagues for their position. If you have considered ways to deal with controversies prior to the meeting, then you will be able to conduct the discussions more effectively.

Physical Arrangement of the Meeting Room

The physical environment can enhance or inhibit the productivity of the meeting. The seating arrangement, the placement of furniture, the shape of the conference table, and your own location in the meeting room can all affect communication patterns. Allowing participants to select their own seats usually helps to establish an open communication atmosphere.

For the most part, faculty, like students, are creatures of habit. They seem to enter the room and sit in the same location for every meeting. This choice can sometimes provide valuable clues about what to expect from a person during a meeting. According to Hunsaker and Alessandra (1986), "Conflict is more likely, for example, between people sitting opposite each other" (p. 192). Usually, faculty choose this seating arrangement in anticipation of conflict or based on past history so that they may carefully view the reactions of a specific colleague. Some faculty members tend to sit close to the department chair because they view that as a power position. This supports the premise that faculty who view themselves as higher in power than others sit closer to the leader or in a location from which they can direct the conversation. Conversely, those who are new to the faculty or believe that their ideas are not valued by others often sit in the back of the room or far away from the leader.

Conducting the Meeting

Faculty meetings can be run in either a formal or informal manner. Formal faculty meetings should strictly adhere to *Robert's Rules of Order*. When this is the case, it is a good idea to have someone designated as the parliamentarian. Informal meetings are less regimented, but should follow some basic established operating policies. If there is not a parliamentarian present, it is the chair's responsibility to maintain order during the meeting. In all types of meetings, it is imperative that a secretary take minutes and maintain an accurate record of discussions and motions that are made and voted upon. Recording names of persons in attendance is one of the first tasks of the secretary. This process also establishes that a quorum is present.

The most important thing to remember once the meeting has begun is to stick to the agenda. Continually reminding the participants about the agenda is necessary when the discussion leads to non-agenda topics. You can reinforce the good points that your faculty are making and offer to place them on the agenda for the next meeting, but you must stay focused on the specific agenda item being discussed.

Meetings normally begin with opening remarks from the chair. These remarks should be positive and concise, and should include a statement about the purpose(s) of the meeting. This would also be the appropriate time to add pre-approved items to the agenda. Adding items to the agenda once it has been distributed is usually not a good idea, but it is sometimes necessary. When these items are added, the chair should be the person to approve the addition, and it should occur before the meeting.

Once you have progressed through the announcement phase of the agenda, you will proceed to those topics on which discussion will be encouraged. Discussion is crucial to good meetings. A good leader will not dominate the discussion, but will instead solicit faculty participation. It is during this phase of the meeting that the leader must maintain neutrality and self-control. Facial expressions and body language can be read easily by faculty; without any verbal interaction, you can inadvertently convey your opinions to the group. Many times, these behaviors inhibit any honest discussion that might occur. The following are items to consider in generating and maintaining control of discussion:

- Ask open-ended questions that can't be answered by yes or no responses.
- Reinforce statements made by participants that are on target with meeting objectives.
- Redirect any questions aimed at the chair to others in the group.
- Carefully use relevant examples out of [your] own experience to encourage the group to think along similar lines.
- Ignore off-target remarks. Discussion only reinforces them.
- Ask questions either of an individual or of the whole group that relate to the task at hand.
- Restate relevant points of the agenda when the discussion veers from objectives.
- Firmly put down participants who dominate any discussion by asking them to let others speak. Acknowledge that you are clear on the point that they were trying to make and ask to hear from other faculty members.
- When an off-the-track subject looms as important, ask the group's opinion as to whether it should be added to the agenda now or at a later meeting.
- As the group moves through the agenda, keep them on track by offering quick summaries (3-M, 1979, p. 88).

If the faculty members come to the meeting prepared for discussion, the items that they present are generally relevant to the specific topic. Even when the agenda has been distributed well in advance, however, many members will come to the meeting unprepared. These faculty will likely direct the discussion away from the main topic and toward a topic that they want to discuss or are more familiar with. It is the leader's responsibility to redirect these individuals' comments in a gentle but firm manner so that the discussion is once again back on track. This situation may occur several times during the discussion, so pay attention to faculty comments and be prepared to redirect the flow of conversation when necessary.

Another problem that arises frequently during discussion is when particular faculty members attempt to dominate the conversation. To deter this, the chair should announce at the beginning of the meeting that each person will be allotted a specified amount of time to speak (e.g., two minutes). It is also important to remember that all faculty should be given the opportunity to express their views during discussion. Once all faculty have had the opportunity to take part in the discussion, those who have already spoken may do so again, but within the established time guidelines. The task of timing the speakers could be assigned to a faculty member, the secretary, or the chair.

At all times during the discussion, the chair must be able to separate ideas from people. This can be difficult at times. Based on previous discussions, the chair may place value judgments on the worthiness of a specific faculty member's ideas. A well-thought-out agenda will help the chair stay focused on the agenda rather than on the personalities involved. While it is important to remain as neutral as possible about who is presenting ideas, you must be prepared for the various types of personalities that inevitably emerge during meetings. As the chair, it is your responsibility to anticipate the types of behaviors that specific attendees will exhibit. If you are aware of potential problems, you will be able to deter some of them. Examples of typical faculty behaviors include:

- The Power-Seeker: The person who attempts to split the group, thereby giving him or herself a higher level of power within the group.
- The Clown or Attention-Seeker: The person who always uses comedy to make a point or draw attention.
- The Dominator: The person who speaks loudly and endlessly about the topic, and is insensitive to other faculty members' ideas, especially if they are not in agreement with his or her own.
- The Facilitator: The person who rewords what others have said and summarizes discussions in an attempt to reach consensus. In this summary, his or her own viewpoint is always represented or singled out as the most appropriate solution to a problem.

Closing the Meeting

When the allocated time for the meeting is over, it is the chair's responsibility to close the meeting. One type of closure is a recommendation. Effective discussions are those that lead to recommendations. Recommendations are not representative of a fixed position, but are reflections of the beliefs of the majority of those who have entered into the discussion. Besides bringing closure to discussions, recommendations tend to represent accomplishment and serve as action items for future meetings.

In most instances, closure should be brief and to the point. If action items have been completed, these should be summarized as a part of the closure. If more discussion is needed, you should acknowledge that it will occur at the next meeting. If faculty have volunteered for or been assigned various duties, those should be stated again, along with the timelines for completion and the format that the final report should take. For example, a faculty member could be appointed to convene an ad hoc committee for the purpose of drafting a written position statement on a specific topic (e.g., the position of the recreation department faculty on increasing the number of distance-learning classes). The concluding remark of the meeting should set the next meeting date and time, which are always subject to change.

Retreats

Action items for the year may be generated for the department at events other than traditional meetings. As a way of beginning an academic year or semester, it has become common for deans and chairs to schedule retreats. Generally, these types of events are held away from campus and may involve one or more days of intense meetings and discussions. Before beginning this type of work-intensive event, many decisions and arrangements must be made. The first of these decisions is to identify the dates and secure the location. Retreats that are held on or near campus may be easier to organize, as they do not require any type of travel or housing arrangements. Off-campus retreats may be preferable, however, in that the participants are physically removed from their daily interruptions.

Deans may schedule retreats for department chairs as a means of enhancing communication between and among the chairs, the dean, and the dean's staff. These types of retreats commonly center on topics such as: developing a strategic plan for the college; the vision of the college; the mission of the college as it relates to the academic structure on campus; preparing for visits from outside accreditation agencies; technology; and distance education. All of these topics will have a direct impact on all departments, and in many cases, they will be affected by budgetary decisions.

Pre-planning the agenda for a retreat is essential. All participants should receive an agenda and other important information in advance. Most of the time, the dean or the chair would be the leader of the total group meetings, but in some instances, it might be beneficial to have an outside facilitator as the person in charge. A highly credentialed professional can serve as a neutral facilitator who will assist the college or department in meeting the purposes of the retreat.

Normally, a department retreat would follow a retreat called by the dean and would center on decisions made during the dean's retreat. For example, once the college mission statement has been developed and approved, departments must then develop or rewrite their mission statement to be in alignment with the college's. A department could also hold a retreat in order to discuss a name change for itself (e.g., "physical education" to "kinesiology" or "exercise science"; "health sciences" to "community health"). In most cases, department retreats will involve a larger group of participants than did the dean's retreat. In order to be successful, the chair should plan for total group meeting and participation time as well as small-group discussions.

Summary

This chapter has included some tips for planning and leading effective meetings and retreats. Whether you are a new chair or a seasoned veteran, you should carefully review your notes following each meeting. By doing so, you will be able to put carry-over items on the next agenda, follow up on any action items, and begin to implement any policy changes that were approved. As with any endeavor, the more experience you have with meetings, the more efficiently they will run.

About the Author

Donna Phillips is a professor in, and chair of, the Physical Education Department at Western Illinois University. She is the past president of the Illinois Association for Health, Physical Education, Recreation, and Dance, and is currently the chairperson-elect of the College and University Administrators Council within the American Association for Active Lifestyles and Fitness.

References

Burleson, C. W. (1990). *Effective meetings: The complete guide.* New York: John Wiley & Sons.

Hunsaker, P. L., & Alessandra, A. J. (1986). *The art of managing people.* New York: Simon & Schuster.

The 3M Meeting Management Team. (1979). *How to run better business meetings.* New York: McGraw-Hill.

12 Effective Faculty Recruiting

Steven W. Smidley, *Assistant Professor and Acting Chairperson, Department of Recreation and Sport Management, Indiana State University*

Barbara A. Passmore, *Professor and Dean, School of Health and Human Performance, Indiana State University*

J. Laurence Passmore, *Professor of Counseling, Indiana State University*

If you walk around, it might not come around.

○━━►○ Barbara Passmore

Faculty-recruitment efforts in health, physical education, recreation, and dance (HPERD) don't have to have these outcomes:

- Search Aborted—Unqualified candidate recommended
- Search Cancelled—Top candidates rejected offer
- Search Re-advertised—Job description misleading
- Search Suspended—Few applicants: poor advertising
- Search Terminated—Called current employer without candidate's permission
- Search Successful, Employee Fired—False credentials

While the authors have collectively observed all of these undesirable outcomes, careful attention to a department's mission, position description, advertising decisions, search-committee selection, reference checks, on-campus interviews, and candidate selection can result in successful recruitment.

Recruitment and the Mission Statement

Recruiting a new colleague involves much more than simply finding another "cog" for the "machine." It is an opportunity for the HPERD administrative unit to realign or renew the direction of the department. Indeed, renewal becomes the theme of the search. As mission statements and accompanying goals are reexamined by the department and the search committee, the role of the departmental within the school/college and the institution is solidified and clarified in the minds of the faculty. In this manner, stakeholders become unified in securing new faculty who complement the department and the various programs within the unit.

In one recent search in the Department of Recreation and Sport Management at Indiana State University (ISU), the faculty were faced with an opportunity to hire either a new chair or a new faculty member. Options were weighed in relation to both departmental and program needs. Since the department supports a common core curriculum with four emphases, discussion of these options was both professional and lively. A decision was made to seek a faculty member who could complement the sports-management curriculum and support the core curriculum of the major.

Recruitment of new HPERD faculty should also be fully contextualized. That is, the department's philosophy, mission, and goals, together with its curricular, research, and instructional needs, should inform the description of the position and specify the required knowledge, skills, and experience. Since new faculty will bring in compatible but different mixtures of these requirements, the department will need to prepare for, and adjust to, various changes. In general, new faculty will likely be supportive of curricular change and resourceful in technological domains. They may also help balance the proportion of junior and senior faculty while fostering political realignment and new levels of expectation.

For example, a recent hire in the ISU Department of Recreation and Sport Management helped the department solve a vexing problem experienced in its computer-applications course. While the search was not specifically geared towards attracting someone who could teach such a course, the search committee's contextualized understanding of the position helped them match the candidate's unique mix of talents to the department's programmatic needs.

Beginning the search process by revisiting the mission of the department provides the context for preparing a thoughtful position description. Indeed, initiating the search process in this manner can help guide the entire process, even up to the mentoring that occurs once the candidate accepts the position and arrives on campus.

Position Description

The position description becomes a written commitment to the implementation of the department's mission, and it gives potential applicants a clear picture of what the position entails. If the description is sufficiently precise, it is quite probable that only those candidates who have high interest in the position and appropriate credentials and talents will apply for the job. Vague or "open" position descriptions typically attract far too many applicants, many with minimal qualifications. The search committee may find it helpful to survey recent position announcements for samples of effective content and wording. A position description should include:

- position title and rank
- minimal qualifications required, including degree
- experience, research interests, and any licensing or certification requirements, if applicable
- responsibilities of the position, including expectations related to teaching, research, and service
- advisement, administration, supervision, thesis direction, and so forth
- information about the department, including its mission, research, enrollment, degree programs, accreditation status, service functions, and number of faculty

- salary and benefits information
- application procedures
- screening dates
- contact information for the department or search committee
- a request for recommendations
- due date.

With respect to the last two items above, several suggestions are offered. References' names, addresses, and telephone numbers are preferable to letters of recommendation. As Schneider (2000) stated, "In academe, some letters really are too good to be true" (p. A17). Letters can be used as an initial resource, but phone contact with references allows the search committee to pose specific questions about a candidate's qualifications in relation to the position description. Typically, more frank answers are solicited in this manner.

A flexible due date is recommended. Due dates should be communicated in a manner that gives the search committee maximum flexibility in their effort to find the most qualified candidates. Using phrases such as "Until the position is filled" or "Applications may not be considered after (a certain date)" provides such flexibility.

In all cases, the position description should be the one document that expresses most clearly the intent and direction of the search. In many institutions of higher education, this description is viewed as a legal document of sorts, representing a contract to fill a position. Therefore, great care must be taken to assure that the statement is prepared in a manner consistent with the procedures of the university while still meeting the needs of the department and accurately describing the position.

Advertising the Position

Once the position description is written, an advertising plan for recruitment should be developed. Appropriate and useful vehicles for advertising a position include: *The Chronicle of Higher Education*, various minority publications, and the listservs, journals, and newsletters of organizations such as the College and University Administrators Council (CUAC), the National Association for Physical Education in Higher Education (NAPEHE), the American Alliance for Health, Physical Education, Recreation, and Dance (AAHPERD), the American Association for Health Education (AAHE), and the National Recreation and Park Association (NRPA). One should then identify the submission deadlines for selected outlets; advertisements should be submitted with sufficient lead time (a minimum of four weeks for most hard-copy publications).

Search-Committee Selection

Well before a search begins, considerable thought must be given to the make-up of the search committee. In some institutions, the procedures for the selection and composition of a search committee are matters of established policy. Whether the committee is appointed or elected, or consists of volunteers, it is important that members understand their role as stakeholders. Each committee member should understand and appreciate the mission and needs of the department and accept the position description.

To ensure diversity, it is useful if the committee has a balanced representation of junior and senior faculty and various minorities. More important, some members should represent the specific discipline called for in the position description. It has also become conventional to include department alumni and respected professionals in the field. Representation from other units or disciplines that complement the mission of the department may be appropriate. Should the HPERD departments have auxiliary units (e.g., dance studios, outdoor recreation facilities, golf courses), representatives from these units could be included on the committee as well. Finally, community agencies that are stakeholders in the discipline could be represented. For example, in the case of a search for a health-education professional, a representative of a local community health or social-service agency could be selected for the committee. While the search committee should represent as many stakeholders as possible, its size needs to be kept to practical limits. The goal here is to form a strong team that represents the interests of the department and that is committed to efficient and effective recruitment.

The committee chair should have prior experience in conducting faculty searches, a good understanding of the university's search and hiring procedures, and a close working relationship with the department chair. The committee chair's responsibilities are to oversee the search, to assure that university policy and procedures are followed, and to direct the committee in the best interests of the department. Other responsibilities of the committee chair include:

- keeping the department chair informed of the progress of the search;
- creating candidate files and updating them as needed;
- notifying candidates of decisions;
- protecting the confidentiality of the candidates; and
- processing all necessary documents in accordance with university policy.

The charge to the committee is prepared and delivered by the department chair. The charge should be given in both written and verbal form. The written version allows the committee to refer to the charge throughout the search process. The charge statement should include:

- the connection between the search and the department's vision;
- a clear description of the position and the required qualifications;
- a reminder to follow the guidelines of confidentiality attendant to the process and to individual candidates;
- a caution to attend to detail in all steps of the search, including university policy, search procedures, and employment law; and
- the expectations of the chair regarding the form and content of the committee recommendations.

The importance of confidentiality should be highlighted. Many a search has been put in jeopardy by the failure of committee members to protect the confidentiality of the process and of individual candidates. Early disclosure of candidate identities or committee decisions can lead to embarrassment at minimum, and perhaps even to dissolution of the search. High-profile positions will attract news-media attention. In these cases, the need for confidentiality will be even more important. The committee chair becomes the official spokesperson for the committee, and only he or she should release information about the search when it is appropriate to do so.

Candidate Materials

A system for review and evaluation of candidate materials should also be developed. Materials should be kept in a secure location; since this is a confidential process, only search-committee members and the chair should have access to the documents. A sign-in/out form should be used to record access to candidate files and to document committee participation. Additional forms should be created for committee members to use in reviewing and evaluating candidates.

After initial review of candidate materials, the committee should sort candidates into two groups: those who are not qualified or no longer under consideration, and those who are qualified. A series of sorting actions may be required, depending on the size of the candidate pool. If the pool is unusually large, a sub-committee can work to reduce it to a manageable size using the desired qualifications for the position. The goal is to reduce the pool to those candidates who most closely match the desired qualifications, all in preparation for the next step: reference checking.

Reference Checks

It is recommended that reference and credential checks take place by phone. Such checks are very important steps in the selection process. Nothing in the candidate's application should be taken for granted or assumed accurate until it is verified. Although this verification is time-consuming and tedious, it is a necessary process. Initially, references provided by the candidate should be contacted for further inquiry. In addition to these references, an effort should be made to identify, with the candidate's permission, other individuals who could provide information about him or her (e.g., HPERD professional colleagues, former employers, or anyone who may be able to speak to the candidate's suitability for the position). The purpose of this expanded reference check is to get feedback about the candidate from as many people as possible. If the committee wishes to contact the candidate's current employer and this individual is not listed as a reference, then they must obtain the candidate's approval; candidates may not want their current employer contacted until they are on the committee's "very short list."

Committee members should work in pairs when contacting references so that there is a witness to each call. If committee members cannot work in pairs, then audio recordings of the reference calls can be made, with the permission of the references.

A set of core questions should be developed for use with each reference. Responses to these questions should be recorded in writing for review by the full committee. Before any questions are asked, references should be given a clear understanding of the requirements of the position in order to best describe the candidate's qualifications.

On-Campus Interviews

The decision to bring a candidate to campus for an interview is a crucial one. Only those candidates who are acceptable for the position should be extended an on-campus interview. This is not the time for "courtesy interviews." Interviewing candidates who are unacceptable is a disservice to both them and the institution; candidates are falsely encouraged, and both they and the institution expend unnecessary time and money.

Attention should be given to the order and the number of candidates invited for on-campus interviews. Search policies and budget constraints may affect these decisions. Whether the most desirable candidate visits campus last or first, comparison of the candidates can best be made if all of the visits are within a one-to-two-week time frame.

In preparation for the on-campus interview, the search committee, in conjunction with the chair, must make meticulous arrangements for travel and for on-campus activities. As Waggaman (1983) stated, "The purpose of the campus interview should be to persuade the candidate to accept a job offer" (p. 41). The visit should include the following individuals and groups:

- dean, associate/assistant dean
- local professionals
- faculty
- staff
- students
- class or research presentation group
- graduate dean
- other stakeholders
- search committee
- realtor

Before the visit, materials about the campus should be sent to each invitee (e.g., catalogues, HPERD curricular information, strategic plans, mission statements, school/department organization charts). A packet from the local chamber of commerce should also be sent to them.

During a meeting before the campus interview, the search committee should create open-ended questions to be asked of each candidate. Their focus should be on the job description. Possible candidate answers should be discussed in the context of the questions. Additionally, the committee should pose questions that the candidate may ask and provide sample answers to these questions. The campus visit procedure should provide some uniformity in assessing candidates and solidify the planning and vision discussed during the initial portions of the search process.

Selecting a Candidate

Upon completion of the on-campus interviews, search-committee discussions should be held as soon as possible. After evaluations have been collected from various sources and reviewed, the committee can begin its own evaluation of the candidates, keeping in mind the position description and departmental mission. The goal of such discussion is to form a recommendation that can be forwarded to the chair in accordance with the policies of the university. The committee should be required to forward a specific number of candidates to the department chair and the dean for review and selection. All forwarded candidates must meet the qualifications for the position and be deemed acceptable by the committee. The actual number of candidates forwarded will depend on the size of the candidate pool and the level of competitiveness for the position. In any case, the committee should be able to reduce the pool to at least two (and no more than four or five) individuals. The forwarded names should *not be ranked* by the committee, however. Instead, recommendations should be accompanied by a narrative describing each candidate's strengths and weaknesses. The recommendations should be presented to the department chair with all committee members attending. This process gives the department chair a full sense of the committee's deliberations.

As the chair and then the dean assess the information offered by the search committee, substantial evaluation of each candidate's compatibility with the vision and planning of the HPERD department must occur. Although no candidate will be a perfect "fit," some strengths are more desirable than others, and some weaknesses are rather inconsequential.

Once the decision is made concerning the individual who best fits the department's mission, vision, and position description, an offer is made to that candidate by either the dean or the department chair. The candidate will no doubt want some time to consider the offer and/or propose a counter-offer. Additional incentives (e.g., moving expenses, research equipment, increased travel money and/or salary) can be offered in order to secure the individual. Once the offer is accepted, the committee chair notifies all applicants that the search has been completed and that a candidate has accepted the position. All files are stored in case of appeals.

Summary

Departments should search, interview, and hire with retention in mind. The culmination of faculty recruitment is not merely the act of hiring a candidate. Retention of strong HPERD faculty is necessary to build strong departments and schools. The work of retention begins at hiring and continues with the welcoming, orientation, and mentoring of a new faculty member. It is the search committee's responsibility to actively support new hires. They must take the lead in welcoming and guiding new faculty.

About the Authors

Steven W. Smidley, assistant professor and acting chairperson of the Department of Recreation and Sport Management at Indiana State University, has conducted personnel searches in the recreation field, for association management, and in higher education.

Barbara A. Passmore, professor and dean in the School of Health and Human Performance at Indiana State University, has been an administrator since 1983 and has chaired many searches during her 32-year history at the institution.

J. Laurence Passmore, professor of counseling at Indiana State University, has also served as chair of the Department of Counseling.

References

Schneider, A. (2000). Why you can't trust letters of recommendation. *Chronicle of Higher Education, 46*(40), A17.

Waggaman, J. S. (1983). *Faculty recruitment, retention, and fair employment: Obligations and opportunities (ASHE-ERIC/Higher Education Research Report no. 2).* Washington, DC: Association for the Study of Higher Education.

13 Faculty Development: Preparing for Change in the 21st Century

Erika Sander, *Assistant Vice Chancellor of Human Resources and Associate Professor of Human Kinetics, University of Wisconsin–Milwaukee*

Anthony Ciccone, *Director of the Center for Instructional and Professional Development and Professor of French, University of Wisconsin–Milwaukee.*

Certainly the freedom to pursue ideas, to raise inconvenient questions, to create an agenda of inquiry that builds on one's imagination and curiosity must be maintained as essential to the work of the professoriate, and these [freedoms have been] identified by new faculty as important. But it is clear...that the notion of professional autonomy has been pressed too far and misappropriated. For some faculty it has become, to use Philip Slater's phrase, 'The pursuit of loneliness.' Collaboration and professional autonomy are not necessarily incompatible; each can benefit from the other. But developing a collaborative organization will require reexamining the relationship between autonomy and responsibility in the faculty career. (Rice, 1996, p. 27)

As R. Eugene Rice suggested, faculty of the 21st century will be working in a changing higher-education environment, one characterized by collaboration, accountability, and, as the Kellogg Commission has challenged, greater engagement. This runs counter to the relative autonomy of faculty work that characterized the campus of the 20th century. Addressing the tension between autonomy and collaboration is critical to developing effective faculty in the 21st century. We have also begun to focus more on student learning and on peer review of teaching. Locke (1995) identified the challenges we face within leisure and health sciences as he explored Boyer's now-acclaimed *Scholarship Reconsidered* model (in Boyer, 1990); specifically, Locke concluded:

In the end, physical educators have no right to ask for parity in rewards. What we deserve is what we can earn in the judgment of our peers—when the playing field of excellence is level for everyone: teachers, discoverers, synthesizers, clinicians, and those who try to use their knowledge in the applications of service. That is the vision we must hold firm, in reconsidering what scholarship means in physical education. (p. 521)

This leads us to frame faculty development in the context of (1) our changing higher-education environment, (2) professional motivations of faculty throughout their career, and (3) faculty roles and rewards. From our experience and that of others, we will provide practical suggestions for addressing faculty development in a variety of contexts (e.g., research and comprehensive universities; primarily undergraduate institutions).

Our Changing Higher-Education Environment

As noted in Rice's opening quote, the basic tension between autonomy and collaboration in faculty work is the key to understanding faculty development. Plater (1995) put it another way, in the context of the currently changing university environment: "[There is] a built-in tension between standardization and individualization, between centralization and decentralization" (p. 27). Christina (2000) explored how the Kellogg Commission's (1999) notion of the engaged university can be incorporated into our fields. He listed 11 ways of promoting engagement, the most pertinent of which to faculty development are: (1) to create learning communities; (2) to enlarge our perspective and definition of scholarship to make it more inclusive; (3) to reexamine faculty roles and work priorities; and (4) to reexamine how faculty are evaluated and rewarded. We would reason that the tension between autonomy and collaboration, centralization and decentralization, is best addressed in unfettered conversation about faculty roles, development, and rewards. That conversation is often best accomplished by exploring the least public, least peer-reviewed faculty role—teaching! As Hutchings and Shulman (1999) have frequently observed, the scholarship of teaching (from the Boyer model) will become credible only when teaching invites peer collaboration; specifically, teaching and student learning must become public, must open themselves to critique and evaluation in a form that others can build on.

While this seems logical and doable, Kraft (2000) has noted that faculty separate their lives into segments (e.g., home, teaching, department, and research) and that "sustained, in-depth conversation about teaching—especially in a public forum—is seen as taking teaching too seriously" (p. 49), especially at the department level. Through campus-wide conversations about teaching and learning, Kraft's university has built well-received learning communities in cross-departmental formats. Unfortunately, some departments have been unable to engage in this sort of discourse because of their disciplinary focus. Kraft reasoned that this is due to faculty members' graduate-school preparation, where the pursuit of knowledge is largely isolated; specifically, scholarly writing is primarily objective, impersonal, and scientific, characterized by dispassionate observation. Teaching, on the other hand, is about feelings, which are "unscientific" and, therefore, not to be taken seriously. Departments continue to focus primarily on objective criteria when evaluating faculty for retention, promotion, tenure, and compensation, thus reinforcing faculty autonomy over collaboration. Departments must begin to engage in conversation about faculty roles, development, and rewards, and about how they will address the autonomy-versus-collaboration tensions that faculty experience throughout their careers.

One way to approach these tensions is to explore the motivations and desires of faculty throughout their careers. We have noted from both the literature and our own work that faculty exhibit the following general characteristics as they prepare for and move through their professorial careers:

The Changing Motivations of Faculty

Graduate Student

- Development of skill set for teaching, research, and service involvement
- Basic grounding for professional development, with solid faculty mentoring

Assistant Professor through Promotion/Tenure

- Wants to develop effective teaching methods
- Wants to develop a research program
- Wants to establish collegial and mentoring relationships that support personal development

Associate Professor through Promotion to Full Professor

- Mature as a teacher; more actively involved with student learning
- Gains stature as a scholar/researcher
- Wants to continue collegial and mentoring relationships; begins to assume mentor role

Mid- through Late Career

- Wants to develop as a mentor, facilitator, leader
- Engages in more scholarly and academic program development
- Assumes one of three generic career paths:
  (1) Academic administration (e.g., dean, provost)
  (2) "Balanced professor" and more of a meta-scholar
  (3) Continued commitment to a visible, acclaimed research program

Retirement Period (assuming there is continued involvement)

- Wants to mentor younger faculty and graduate students
- Wants to continue teaching part-time
- Wants to be more reflective, analytic (a "resident expert")

Obviously, the way in which faculty prioritize work at different stages of their careers varies, as it should. Several themes emerge: (1) the desire for autonomy to develop as a scholar, (2) the desire to be an effective teacher, and (3) the desire for collegial interaction and mentoring relationships. These themes should inform any efforts at faculty development. Explicitly or implicitly, faculty want both autonomy and collaborative relationships that spin around all three areas of faculty responsibility—teaching, research, and professional service.

Faculty have also been asked to compare what they believe their duties to be with what their institution expects from them. Diamond and Adam (1998) conducted a series of studies in which they sought to determine

Faculty Roles and Rewards

how faculty, department chairs, and deans perceived the balance between research and undergraduate teaching at their institutions (N=49, research and doctoral, national sample). Findings in 1991-92 were remarkably consistent; most of the faculty and administrators felt that their institutions *should* favor a balance between undergraduate teaching and research, though they perceived a strong institutional emphasis on research. In a 1996 follow-up study with 11 institutions from the original sample, several important trends were noted:

- Priorities are changing at many research institutions, with stronger support for a balance between research and teaching.
- The study participants perceived that their institutions were placing greater importance on teaching.
- The percentage of study participants reporting a strong personal emphasis on research declined.
- In open-ended comments, respondents reported that while institutional rhetoric has changed, policies and practices for promotion, tenure, and merit pay continue to reward research over undergraduate teaching.

Yet these findings stem primarily from research/doctoral institutions. In dialogue with colleagues in the American Association for Higher Education (AAHE) "Faculty Roles and Rewards" forum who represent comprehensive and undergraduate-centered universities, we noted that their institutional cultures tend to emphasize teaching more than research. Further, these colleagues have indicated that scholarly work, while not as critical as in research institutions, is viewed by the professoriate as a critical adjunct to teaching. They also seek a better balance between teaching and scholarly work. The key factor that seemed to permeate the "Faculty Roles and Rewards" cauldron of the 1990s was the perceived, if not real, disconnection between faculty roles and reward systems, most especially those related to tenure, promotion, and annual merit compensation.

With this in mind, we will present examples of "best practices" for faculty development that address this disconnection within the context of the changing higher-education landscape of the 21st century. It is critical that the academy position itself competitively as it addresses the expectations of our very change-oriented society, and that it pursues this with an appropriate balance between student learning, scholarly work, and professional service. Finally, there must be an institutional commitment (strategic and fiscal) to the development and support of faculty and all human resources, including teaching and research assistants and support staff. Development programs must in turn be responsive to institutional initiatives.

"Best Practices" for Faculty Development

The Faculty-Development Plan. At the outset, academic units and campus communities need to engage in conversation to clarify their various initiatives. At the departmental level, the conversation should focus on the relationships between teaching, student learning, research, scholarship, and professional service/outreach.

Best Practice #1 (for chairs): Set aside 15 minutes at every department meeting for a "show and tell," where a colleague or two present and discuss how they have connected teaching and student learning with their scholarly work.

Again, both the literature and our own experience strongly suggest that faculty want to engage in teaching and student learning with more vigor. They also appreciate the connection between teaching, scholarly work, and professional service, the balance of which tends to shift throughout one's career. Finally, the way that faculty duties are operationalized, developed, and rewarded is of major concern to them. Consequently, it should also be an institutional concern.

Faculty and instructional staff should also be expected to develop annual workload and development plans that include teaching, scholarship, and service components. To facilitate the creation of realistic Faculty-Development Plans (FDPs), departmental workload policies should respond to changing forms of faculty work (namely, teaching, advising, research, scholarship, and professional service/outreach) throughout a faculty member's career. Faculty rewards (e.g., annual compensation adjustments or merit pay) typically flow from this peer-review process.

Best Practice #2 (for chairs): Make sure that faculty workload policies are annually reviewed and approved by faculty; FDPs should be developed, updated, and reviewed annually.

Best Practice #3 (for deans): Review and approve faculty workload policies; receive, review, and file all FDPs.

Co-author Ciccone has devoted much of his professional career to faculty-development programs, especially in teaching and student learning. When Ciccone first began his career as both a faculty member and a faculty developer, a former vice chancellor outlined for him what was at that time the prevailing wisdom in career advancement. "Now that you've earned a PhD in a specialized area and found a position at an institution similar to where you earned it, pursue your research interests and aspire to teaching your area of specialty to highly motivated graduate students interested in being just like you." It is astonishing to think how different most current faculty careers are from that "ideal," if indeed they ever reflected it. At all points in their careers, faculty are asked to play many roles, to teach a wide variety of courses, and to understand and incorporate a plethora of pedagogical and curricular enhancements.

Faculty-development initiatives, whether within a department or institution-wide, have always been designed to respond to the multiple roles that faculty must play and to prepare faculty for these roles. For example, workshops on active learning, instructional technology, and effective lesson design have helped innumerable instructors meet their student-learning goals (and improve their student evaluations). As faculty roles continue to evolve, however, departments and institutions have had to reconsider the "workshop" response. The emphasis on collaboration, accountability, and greater engagement in the overall life of the department and the institution, outlined earlier, requires a more sophisticated integration of individual and program needs. This understanding has led many departments and institutions to design long-term initiatives that involve many faculty at the same time, each contributing from his or her strengths and gaining from the experience of colleagues.

In order to involve as many faculty as possible in these efforts, many departments and institutions have embraced a developmental model. This model proposes that faculty have different needs, goals, and abilities at different stages in their careers and, thus, that they will be more effective in certain capacities than in others. Our experience in professional development has led us to believe that faculty pass through four stages during the course of their career:

1. A new assistant professor, concerned most with balancing teaching and scholarship and making the classroom an effective and efficient place for learning.
2. A tenured professor, re-examining possibilities and priorities, identifying new paths, and developing new expertise.
3. A full professor, identifying ways to make lasting contributions in areas that matter most.
4. A retired (emeritus) professor, continuing one of these contributions.

At any given time, a department and institution has individuals at each of these stages. Although this may seem to complicate the design of faculty-development programs, it actually simplifies the task, because the expertise of faculty at one stage often reflects the needs and desires of faculty at other stages. The trick, then, lies in bringing these individuals together. What types of programs work best under this developmental philosophy and in the context of the tension between autonomy and collaboration? Following are some examples.

Curriculum Development. New faculty are often hired with the expectation that they will design new courses or update courses taught by faculty who have recently left or retired. Typically, curriculum development takes place in isolation, as much out of respect for faculty autonomy and expertise as out of the difficulty in imagining a collaborative model. The result is often a series of courses with little, if any, articulation. Departments miss a valuable developmental opportunity by operating in this way. A better model, to use a concept proposed by Bass (1999), would be to "problematize" the task for the entire department.

> Best Practice #4 (for chairs): Graduate students, assistant professors, and faculty from other related departments should meet to ask, and tentatively answer, questions of content, assignments, and assessment, perhaps with an outside facilitator.

In the course of the discussion, members reveal what is important to them in teaching, thus laying the groundwork for future collaboration. Graduate students and new faculty begin to learn the ropes, experienced faculty get to share their expertise, and the entire group gets a course that better expresses the department's mission. Moreover, each member gets to contribute from his or her strengths, avoiding the pitfalls of the "deficit" (or remediation) model of professional development.

> Best Practice #5 (or chairs): Specific projects include faculty mentoring of graduate students in syllabus development and group design of core courses (perhaps team-taught, one of the best developmental contexts available to departments) and courses for new freshmen and last-semester seniors.

Understanding and improving student learning. The deficit model of professional development often involves defining what individuals can't do, or could do better, in the classroom. Within this model, departments often counsel new faculty to become "adequate" teachers, with the understanding that they will work on their deficiencies after tenure. Not only does this stance foster mediocrity, it also assumes that those who have tenure have reached a higher level of teaching prowess. Fostering a climate that focuses on understanding and improving student learning can help departments avoid these pitfalls and provide opportunities that are developmentally appropriate and professionally valuable. New faculty, for example, need to become efficient and effective (not fast and adequate) teachers. The best way to do this is to learn techniques for finding out when students are or are not understanding the material, aside from the results of midterms or finals.

> Best Practice #6 (for chairs): Learn about and encourage the use of techniques such as the one-minute paper, exit pass, or Brookfield's Critical Incident Questionnaire in order to provide relatively quick access to student learning and to help new faculty target particular difficulties with the content and processes of their courses.

Such techniques create a climate of shared inquiry (with students and other colleagues) about student learning that increases the likelihood of further collaboration.

Mid-to-late-career faculty are often ready and willing to take this type of investigation to the next level. If new faculty are interested in efficient responses to the learning issues of students right in front of them, more experienced faculty are often interested in sharing the expertise they have acquired in pursuing such questions over the years. Pairing the two groups is often quite fruitful, as new faculty provide fresh perspectives on old issues and experienced faculty help contextualize, and often reduce, the apparent seriousness of the problem. In some cases, experienced faculty are also ready to engage in valuable scholarship concerning teaching and learning; that is, they are capable of examining student learning by designing and implementing studies whose results could be built upon by others within and outside the discipline.

> Best Practice #7 (for chairs and deans): Implement faculty mentoring programs built around teaching. Encourage reciprocal (peer) class observation and discussion. Provide grants for teaching scholars to design and implement research projects on teaching.

By using collaborative approaches focusing on student learning and curriculum development, departments can provide their faculty with a non-threatening forum for developing as facilitators of student learning.

Research/scholarship and professional service. Up until recently, development of young faculty at the departmental level has been a primary, autonomous, and very public developmental endeavor. The challenge for the 21st century is to address both autonomy (self-development) and collaboration (the need to work with others, be critiqued, be affirmed, and develop). For example, active mentoring of young scholars is critical.

Best Practice #8 (for chairs): Senior department faculty, as well as non-departmental faculty with scholarly affinity, should actively mentor new faculty to provide formative as well as summative developmental input. Non-tenured faculty should have written scholarly plans (as part of the FDP) that focus on outputs.

Collaborative scholarly work is to be encouraged, where appropriate, such that the faculty member's collaborative role enhances his or her individual development.

Best Practice #9 (for chairs and deans): Younger faculty should be encouraged and supported in the dissemination of their scholarly outputs within national, peer-reviewed forums.

Their research programs should exhibit a clear "line of inquiry," sensitive to various dimensions of scholarly work (e.g., basic through applied research). Funded grant and contract activity that supports the line of research should be supported and mentored.

The challenge of time management. Currently, productive scholarly programs quite often have a direct link with action-oriented community programs (e.g., fitness programs, athletic training services, programs for senior citizens). These service involvements are often time-intensive, taking away from the balance required to develop as a faculty member. This is where senior faculty are most helpful, since time-management is a learned skill.

Best Practice #10 (for chairs): Mentors of younger faculty should actively facilitate the prioritization of professional (as well as personal) time in order to maximize development. Mentors can take on the more administrative tasks, freeing the younger faculty members to focus on developing applied research plans that serve two important purposes: they should (1) provide accountability (assessment) of program effectiveness, and (2) develop the young scholar (supporting both individual and collaborative needs).

For the more basic research scholar, the opportunity exists to connect the laboratory with the field, as the more applied researcher reaches back to the parent disciplines—a "win/win" configuration.

Summary

We have now come full circle. Starting with the tension between autonomy and collaboration in faculty work, we explored the changing nature of the academy, faculty work, and faculty roles and rewards. We then explored how development programs might respond and use collaborative approaches in open, project-oriented forums. Specific program examples involved terminology that may not be familiar to all readers. We strongly encourage using resources such as Diamond (1994, 1995) and the AAHE and Carnegie Foundation web sites (see "Web Resources") for clarification. If your campus has a faculty/staff-development administrator, seek out that person to help both you and your department. Faculty development is most effective at the departmental level, and when it is characterized by open, public, and collegial engagement of faculty that focuses on real issues such as student learning, scholarly development, and professional service. The challenge is to build on the natural inclinations of faculty, who want to be engaged, work in all roles, and be rewarded for their efforts based on productive, peer-reviewed outcomes.

About the Authors

Erika Sander is assistant vice chancellor of human resources and an associate professor of human kinetics at the University of Wisconsin-Milwaukee.

Anthony Ciccone is Director of the Center for Instructional and Professional Development and a professor of French at this same institution.

Sander and Ciccone collectively have over 30 years of leadership experience in faculty-development programs.

References

Boyer, E. L. (1990). *Scholarship reconsidered: Priorities of the professoriate.* Princeton, NJ: The Carnegie Foundation for the Advancement of Teaching.

Bass, R. (1999). The scholarship of teaching: What's the problem? *Inventio* [On-line], *1*(1). Available: http://www.doiiit.gmu.edu/Archives/feb98/rbass.htm

Christina, R. W. (2000). Advancing engagement in kinesiology and physical education. *Quest, 52*(3), 316-329.

Diamond, R. M. (1994). *Serving on promotion and tenure committees.* Boston: Anker.

Diamond, R. M. (1995). *Preparing for promotion and tenure review.* Boston: Anker.

Diamond, R. M., & Adam, B. E. (1998). *Changing priorities at research universities: 1991-1996.* Syracuse, NY: Syracuse University Center for Change in Higher Education.

Hutchings, P., & Shulman, L. S. (1999). The scholarship of teaching—New elaborations, new developments. *Change, 31*(5), 11-15.

Kellogg Commission on the Future of State and Land-Grant Universities. (1999). *Returning to our roots: The engaged institution.* Washington, DC: National Association of State Universities and Land-Grant Colleges.

Kraft, R. G. (2000). Teaching excellence and the inner life of faculty. *Change, 32*(3), 48-52.

Locke, L. F. (1995). An analysis of prospects for changing faculty roles and rewards: Can scholarship be reconsidered? *Quest, 47,* 506-524.

Plater, W. M. (1995). Future work—Faculty time in the 21st century. *Change, 27*(3), 22-33.

Rice, R. E. (1996). *Making a place for the new American scholar.* Washington, DC: American Association for Higher Education.

Web Resources

American Association for Higher Education (AAHE) (www.aahe.org)—AAHE is a major force in higher education. From the web site's home page, visit the "AAHE Bulletin" (under "Publications") for timely articles and other links of interest.

The Carnegie Foundation for the Advancement of Teaching (www.carnegiefoundation.org)—The Foundation's CASTL (Carnegie Academy for the Scholarship of Teaching and Learning) program is available at this site. First read the "President's Message," wherein Lee S. Shulman provides background on the CASTL and other Carnegie initiatives.

http://www.uwm.edu/Dept/Acad_Aff/FMP/faculty1.htm—This is the site for professional-development programs at the University of Wisconsin–Milwaukee. Links are provided to various professional-development programs within the University of Wisconsin system.

14 Evaluating Faculty

Alan C. Lacy, *Professor and Chair, Department of Health, Physical Education, and Recreation, Illinois State University*

The process is often as important as the product.

⚬═══⚬ Alan C. Lacy

Virtually every institution of higher education has some type of faculty-evaluation system. In order to maintain or improve their status on campus, it is important that academic units in health, kinesiology, and leisure studies (HKLS) use faculty-evaluation systems that are thoughtfully conceived, well-constructed, and thorough. One basic purpose of evaluation is to provide feedback to faculty about how well they are performing their professional responsibilities so that they can take steps to improve their performance. Inevitably, evaluations must serve as the basis for personnel decisions as well.

Evaluating faculty is a major component of virtually every HKLS administrator's workload. It is one of the chair's most difficult and important responsibilities. No other activity holds the same potential for strengthening or weakening faculty morale and productivity. Given the critical importance of this activity, it is crucial to have an effective faculty-evaluation system in place. This system should be comprehensive enough to provide fair and equitable evaluations, yet not so burdensome that it takes an excessive amount of both faculty and administrators' time to operate.

A sound faculty-evaluation program must be designed according to the current best practices and scholarship in this area. Despite the fact that there is lively debate among faculty about appropriate evaluation, there are also broad areas of consensus about it. Some notable works include books by Centra (1993), Braskamp and Ory (1994), Miller (1987), and Arreola (1995). Cashin (1996) suggested that among those knowledgeable of the literature and experienced in the field, there is as much as a 90-percent agreement about the general guidelines for faculty evaluation. These areas of agreement should be reflected in the design of any evaluation program. Thus, the purpose of this chapter is to briefly describe these areas of agreement and provide sources from which readers can get more detailed information as needed.

General Planning Guidelines

The following general guidelines should provide the foundation for making reasoned decisions in planning a faculty-evaluation system for HKLS units.

Base the evaluation system on a common set of values. Arreola (1995) pointed out that no single evaluation system can be successfully applied to all faculty groups. The system should be based on the values of those who intend to use it. These values must be determined and expressed in a way that allows them to be consistently applied in the evaluation process. Without such criteria, evaluation is impossible. The basic context for these criteria is the mission of the institution, which should inform the goals of unit.

Allow 18-to-24 months to fully develop and implement an evaluation system. In developing evaluation systems, departments must systematically gather faculty input. Faculty need to see that their input is valued as an integral part of the goals that underlie their performance criteria. Significant involvement by faculty in the development of an evaluation system will help them accept and take ownership of it. Make certain that enough time is allotted in the development process for faculty discussion before, during, and after the implementation of any system. A new system can take as long as two years to implement. The timeframe may be shorter when a department is simply modifying its system, but it will still take longer than is expected. The developmental process should not be rushed. There is value in discussion and debate. The process can be about changing traditions, values, and attitudes as well, and it is likely that these changes will be accompanied by a wide range of emotions among faculty. Thus, open and lengthy communication should be expected. Even given extensive communication with faculty, however, administrators should still expect resistance. This resistance can be grounded in factors such as: the implication of incompetence that is sometimes associated with evaluation efforts; doubts by faculty that evaluators are competent and trustworthy; or anxiety over increased accountability.

Make certain that administrative support is present. Administrative support is critical for the successful implementation or modification of an evaluation system. Without strong support from administrators, it is unlikely that an effective system can be established.

Integrate both formative and summative assessment into the faculty-evaluation system. An evaluation system should integrate two distinct, but connected, aspects: formative and summative assessment. To do one without the other produces a less effective system. One purpose of any faculty-evaluation system is to provide valid, summative information regarding the quality of faculty performance at all levels and across all disciplinary areas. These data should be the primary criteria used for promotion, tenure, and performance evaluations.

Another purpose of an evaluation program is to provide formative direction for faculty improvement efforts. Annual performance evaluations should not exist separately from a faculty-development program. Evaluation procedures and reports should provide information about a faculty member's areas of strength and needed improvement, and any faculty-development programs should be related to this process.

Evaluate faculty performance in a fair and consistent manner. In order to prevent over-reliance on subjective representations of individuals' performance, an evaluation system must use reliable data-collection methods and clear criteria for interpretations and judgments. It is the primary role of the administration to ensure the integrity of this process. It should be recognized that no system is entirely objective. Arreola (1995) wrote, "True objectivity in a faculty-evaluation system is a myth" (p. 2). Subjective professional judgment of colleagues, administrators, students, and others is a necessary part of such systems. The goal of an effective system is to reduce this subjectivity, not eliminate it.

As much as possible, interpret the data and make resultant personnel decisions at the departmental level. The primary authority to interpret data from faculty evaluations lies with the individual faculty member and his or her department. There are many complex factors involved in the interpretation of this information, particularly in relation to the educational character and mission of each department. Within reason, the evaluation system must be responsive to the individual's and the department's priorities, norms, and positions. Because individual departments have the appropriate disciplinary expertise and the opportunity to observe faculty performance on a firsthand basis, evaluation systems should allow personnel decisions to be made primarily at this level.

Link merit pay, tenure, promotion, and faculty evaluation and development. Personnel decisions should be based directly on faculty evaluation and development data that have been collected in a systematic, predictable, and fair way, and faculty should understand how these decisions are reached. If this is not done, then the evaluation program is doomed to failure. The expectations for earning tenure should be strongly correlated to promotion and pay raises. A probationary faculty member should not be able to receive merit raises without making adequate progress toward earning tenure. Furthermore, faculty-development programs should be geared to facilitate performance as defined in the evaluation system.

Perform pilot evaluations to test the efficacy of your system. Whatever system is adopted, there will be unforeseen problems that need to be addressed. Use your proposed system to collect data from volunteer faculty. Given the results of this trial run, necessary changes can be made. These data should not be used for evaluation purposes, though.

Conduct periodic reviews of the evaluation system. An evaluation system should be considered a dynamic instrument for assessing faculty performance. Given that circumstances in higher education are constantly changing, provisions should be made for modifications of the system. Any faculty-evaluation system is necessarily complex and sensitive. It will need to be reviewed regularly to ensure that it remains effective. A new system should be reviewed annually for the first few years and then at regular intervals (e.g., every three to five years) after it is established.

Guidelines for Defining Faculty Performance

Defining faculty performance areas in HKLS units is a crucial step toward developing an effective faculty-evaluation system. The following guidelines are suggested to facilitate this process.

Define major areas of faculty performance at your institution. In most HKLS units at four-year institutions, teaching, scholarship, and service are identified as the three primary areas of faculty performance. At community colleges, the areas of teaching and service are often emphasized. Some institutions may include separate performance categories for advisement, professional development, and administrative duties. It is important that faculty clearly understand what these areas are. Time should be spent determining what the faculty areas are and itemizing faculty activities under these broad categories. For instance, in the teaching area, activities such as regular instruction, curriculum development, supervision of internships, and work on thesis committees would typically be included.

Reach consensus on how the major faculty performance areas should be weighted. Assuming that the major performance areas at your institution are teaching, scholarship, and service, are they weighted equally? Are there greater expectations for teaching than for scholarship and service? If so, they should be weighted at appropriate percentages during evaluation. Faculty must have input in these decisions and know the relative weightings of the identified performance areas. Obviously, the specific mission and values of the institution will impact these weightings.

Some flexibility should be provided in the weightings. Cashin (1996) stated that the use of a singular evaluation system for all faculty virtually guarantees that it will be unfair to everyone. Creating multiple evaluative options can provide the flexibility needed to account for changing faculty roles within the department. Faculty members' roles can change at various stages of their career. Typically, young tenure-track faculty have a greater desire to establish a scholarly line of inquiry and develop their teaching skills than to provide professional service. After receiving tenure and promotion, some faculty may be granted administrative duties or special assignments that benefit the department and, therefore, have heavier service expectations. Faculty-evaluation systems should be designed for consistency, but elements of flexibility can benefit both the faculty and the department. For example, a flexible system could be set up in which teaching is weighted at 40 percent, scholarship at 20 percent, and service at 20 percent, with the remaining 20 percent to be assigned to one of the areas after faculty individually consult with the chair. Another model could provide ranges in each of three areas (e.g., teaching weighted from 30 to 50 percent, scholarship from 30 to 50 percent, and service from 20 to 40 percent). Individual faculty and the chair would come to some agreement as to what the relative amounts would be.

Divide each faculty performance area into major components. Each faculty performance area contains a lengthy list of activities that faculty perform. Somewhat like a statistical factor analysis procedure, these activities should be grouped to develop components of each performance area. For instance, the service area might have components such as departmental service, college and university service, community service, and service to professional organizations. Each of these components could be weighted differently. At this stage, having candid conversations about how service activities are valued is imperative. Ultimately, compromises must be reached as to how each of the identified components is to be weighted.

Arreola (1995) provided an excellent discussion of the components of teaching. He identified them as content expertise, instructional-delivery skills, instructional-design skills, and course-management skills. Asking faculty how they would weight these four components will ensure a lively debate. A task force on assessing and improving instruction at Indiana State University developed a report that may provide further valuable insight about the evaluation of teaching. This report (Center for Teaching and Learning, Indiana State University, 1998) suggested six components of teaching and provided ranges for weighting so that individual departments would have the flexibility to determine their own weightings. The identified components of teaching (and their suggested ranges) were content knowledge (10 to 25 percent), course design (15 to 25 percent), instructional delivery (15 to 30 percent), instructional relationships (15 to 30 percent), course management (5 to 10 percent), and professional development (10 to 25 percent). Teaching environments vary greatly in HKLS. There are instructional settings in traditional classrooms, laboratories, and activity environments. Additionally, some classes are delivered through various distance-education formats. Despite this wide variety of teaching environments, the institution's six established instructional components are foundational to all types of teaching. It is possible to adjust the weightings for these components in the different teaching environments, if desired. Consideration for faculty working with students on independent studies, theses, dissertations, and professional-practice supervision must also be factored into the teaching evaluation.

Given the wide variety of expectations at different institutions in the area of scholarship, it is very important to go through the same process of developing the major components and their weightings in this area. Faculty members need to know what is valued in scholarship. If a focused line of data-based research in nationally recognized, refereed publications is needed to receive tenure, this criterion should be clear to incoming faculty members. If attracting external funding thought grant-writing is a requisite for tenure and promotion, this fact should be reflected in the component weights.

After sufficient time has been spent by faculty and administrators to clearly define and weight faculty performance areas and the components of each area, attention must be given to the assessment sources that provide the data for faculty evaluations. An effective faculty-evaluation model relies on procedures that assure the collection of reliable, valid, and adequate information. Because faculty performance involves many dimensions, it is best to gather information from a number of sources (e.g., students, peers, administrators, self-assessments). Sources should provide information about those areas of faculty performance with which they are most familiar. The following guidelines should be considered when weighing assessment sources.

Include student input, particularly in the area of teaching. Students are the group most directly affected by the quality of faculty teaching. As first-hand observers in the classes, students are in the best position to evaluate specific and critical aspects of a faculty member's teaching practices. They are the only individuals who regularly observe us in action, and it is for

Guidelines for Assessing Faculty Performance

fit that we teach. Student feedback in the faculty-evaluation system can be in formative or summative form. Techniques for evaluation can range from the very formal to the more informal. At the formal end of the spectrum are the summative evaluation instruments seen at most institutions of higher learning. Informal techniques can serve as valuable formative tools (e.g., student journals, open-ended questions, unsigned letters to fictitious friends who are thinking of taking the class) (Murray, 1995). Many of the formative evaluation techniques should be implemented after students have had enough time to become familiar with a teacher's style, but no later than midterm, to allow for mid-semester modifications. Formal student evaluations given at the end of the semester are typically used for summative purposes, but they can be used in formative ways as well. Such student ratings are one of the most common features of faculty-evaluation systems. Seldin (1993) reported that more than 85 percent of all faculty-evaluation systems regularly used student ratings in the early 1990s.

Unfortunately, student ratings are often the *only* component used to evaluate teaching. Given that this information is sometimes used to justify negative personnel decisions, it is understandable that student ratings are not met with universal acclaim from faculty! This over-reliance on student perspectives has led to many myths and misconceptions about student ratings in general It is critical that any such instrument be reliable and valid and provide meaningful feedback that can be used for making improvements. Because locally developed rating forms may not possess the necessary psychometric qualities of reliability and validity, it is generally a good idea to adopt an existing form rather than developing one from scratch (Arreola, 1995). Cashin (1995) and Arreola both provide excellent summaries of the research examining variables related to student ratings. Finally, because students typically are not firsthand observers of the scholarship and service efforts of faculty, they should have little or no input in the evaluation of these performance areas.

Consider the advantages and disadvantages of peer evaluation in assessing the teaching, scholarship, and service areas. Peer assessment in the area of teaching has both advantages and disadvantages. It is certainly advantageous that colleagues are familiar with departmental goals, programs, and priorities, and that they are usually from the same discipline. However, this type of familiarity can also have negative consequences resulting from bias due to previous evaluations, personal relationships, and peer pressure (Arreola, 1995). Collegial review takes two basic forms: classroom visitation and review and critique of course materials. These types of review have traditionally been used for both formative and summative assessment. Researchers have reported that visitation ratings have less inter-rater reliability and a greater bias toward leniency than student ratings (Braskamp, Brandenbury, & Ory, 1984; Centra, 1975). Findings like these make the validity of peer-visitation ratings highly debatable; researchers suggest that visitation is more appropriate for faculty-development activities than for summative evaluation.

It is also suggested that colleagues can provide valuable, reliable, and valid assessments of course materials such as examinations, syllabi, course assignments, and instructional media (Kulik & McKeachie, 1975). Colleagues can also play an integral role in evaluating scholarly efforts. Typically, they are familiar with the field and the rigor and prestige of various conferences and professional journals. Colleagues outside of the institution can also be used in this area. If this option is chosen, care must be taken to ensure that the external reviewers understand the institutional and departmental expectations for scholarship. Similarly, peers can effectively evaluate service contributions. External colleagues can be valuable assessment sources regarding service outside the department.

Ensuring fair and equitable procedures in the faculty-evaluation process is the primary role of administrators. The dean should ensure that faculty development and faculty evaluation are carried out in fair, equitable, and systematic ways at the departmental and school/college level. Because the dean is seldom a firsthand observer of teaching and is likely outside the discipline of the faculty member, she or he should not be directly involved with the assessment of teaching, scholarship, or service.

A primary role of the chair is to oversee departmental procedures for both summative and formative evaluation. The chair must work to build trust and integrity into these ongoing processes. As a source for evaluation, the chair has many of the same advantages and disadvantages as departmental colleagues. Generally, it is logistically impossible for chairs to visit the classes of all faculty members enough times to reliably evaluate them. As with colleague visitations, occasional observations by the chair can be biased by personal relationships, common values, favored teaching methods, and so forth. Class visitations for professional-development purposes may be appropriate, but they are problematic for summative purposes.

In most cases, chairs should be able to adequately evaluate course design and content expertise. Moreover, the chair is in the best position to evaluate the course-management components of teaching (e.g., textbook orders, holding class, office hours, turning in grades on time). Chairs can also have particular insights into the service and administrative contributions of faculty. Similar to faculty colleagues, the chair can contribute to evaluation of scholarship in many instances as well. Nevertheless, the principal characteristics for chairs who oversee faculty evaluations should be impartiality, vigilant protection of faculty rights, and active support of faculty-development efforts.

Combine reflection, self-assessment, and input from other sources for effective use of self-evaluation as an assessment source. Although self-evaluation of performance is necessarily subjective, it can result in performance improvements when accompanied by reflection, self-assessment, and input from other sources. The strength of self-evaluation is that faculty are most likely to act on data that they themselves have collected. The various means of gathering information to assess performance relative to personal needs and goals may be used as an ongoing program of continuous formative assessment. The weakness of the process is that most faculty tend to rate themselves higher than do students and colleagues (Arreola, 1995).

Arreola (1995) identified several conditions for effective use of self-evaluation. First, instructors need to understand precisely how the information is going to be used in order to feel confident and secure in the process. The exact form and substance of the self-evaluation would likely differ for faculty at different stages of their career. Faculty need to have skills in identifying goals and collecting appropriate data. Chairs should facilitate this process, and the teaching-learning center found at many institutions should be a valuable resource in providing this type of training.

Effective self-evaluation requires self-reflection and self-assessment. Further, it should be used in conjunction with administrator/colleague observations and student feedback to determine if the instructor's self-perceptions of performance are consistent with more objective observations. Differences in perceptions can be used to target weaknesses and strengths that are integral to the improvement of faculty performance. Ideally, faculty will reflect thoughtfully upon their performance and compare this self-reflection with more objective perceptions of colleagues and students to modify their efforts as needed.

Weight assessment sources appropriately. While it is important to use multiple data sources for faculty evaluation, it is not necessary or desirable for all of them to be weighted equally. As much as possible, the primary assessment sources should be in a position for firsthand observation of performance. When the main performance areas are subdivided into components, it is possible that the various data sources can be weighted differently in the various component areas. For some components, it may be inappropriate to use a particular assessment source. For example, if it proves impossible for the chair to make sufficient classroom observations, then she or he should not rate the instructional-delivery component. Students, on the other hand, should have greater input in that component, but little or no weighting in the content expertise area. One teaching evaluation model (Center, 1998) suggested the following ranges for the various assessment sources: students (25 to 45 percent), peers (25 to 45 percent), chair (10 to 25 percent), and self-evaluation (5 to 10 percent). These percentages are suggested specifically for the teaching area and are intended to allow departmental flexibility in determining the exact weighting of the assessment sources. Space does not allow further detail as to how this model can work. The task force that recommended this system based it on suggestions in Arreola (1995). Thus, the reader is directed to these sources for further information. Similar assessment models for service and scholarship can be designed with appropriate source weightings (e.g., student sources would not be appropriate in these performance areas unless the students were in a position to be firsthand observers).

Summary

The purpose of this chapter has been to briefly summarize areas of agreement in the current scholarship on faculty-evaluation procedures in HKLS, and to provide sources from which readers can get more detailed information as needed. The trend of increased accountability has been present in higher education for quite some time and is not likely to diminish in the foreseeable future. The development or modification of a faculty-evaluation system is thus a necessary, albeit time-consuming, venture. To rush this process invites failure. It is hoped that the guidelines suggested in this chapter will prove valuable to those charged with planning and implementing faculty-evaluation systems in HKLS academic units.

About the Author

Alan C. Lacy, professor and chair in the Department of Health, Physical Education, and Recreation at Illinois State University, has been in higher education for 18 years, the last six years as a chair.

Arreola, R. (1995). *Developing a comprehensive faculty-evaluation system.* Boston: Anker.

Braskamp, L., Brandenbury, D., & Ory, J. (1984). *Evaluating teaching effectiveness: A practical guide.* Beverly Hills, CA: Sage.

Braskamp, L., & Ory, J. (1994). *Assessing faculty work: Enhancing individual and institutional performance.* San Francisco: Jossey-Bass.

Cashin, W. (1995). *Student ratings of teaching: The research revisited. IDEA paper no. 32.* Manhattan, KS: Center for Faculty Evaluation and Development, Kansas State University.

Cashin, W. (1996). *Developing an effective faculty rating system. IDEA paper no. 33.* Manhattan, KS: Center for Faculty Evaluation and Development, Kansas State University.

Center for Teaching and Learning, Indiana State University. (1998). *Task force report on assessing and improving teaching and learning at Indiana State University* [On-line]. Available: http://web.indstate.edu/ctl/rept/imp.htm

Centra, J. (1975). Colleagues as raters of classroom instruction. *Journal of Higher Education, 46,* 327-337.

Centra, J. (1993). *Reflective faculty evaluation.* San Francisco: Jossey-Bass.

Kulik, J., & McKeachie, W. (1975). The evaluation of teachers in higher education. In F. N. Kerlinger (Ed.), *Review of research in education, 3* (pp. 210-240). Itasca, IL: Peacock.

Miller, R. (1987). *Evaluating faculty for promotion and tenure.* San Francisco: Jossey-Bass.

Murray, J. (1995). *Successful faculty development and evaluation: The complete teaching portfolio (ASHE-ERIC Higher Education Report no. 8).* Washington, DC: Graduate School of Education and Human Development, George Washington University.

Seldin, P. (1993). How colleges evaluate professors—1983 v. 1993. *AAHE Bulletin,* October, 6-12.

References

SECTION III

Building a Financial Base

15 Building a Financially Stable and Functioning Administrative Unit

Tony A. Mobley, *Professor and Dean, School of Health, Physical Education, and Recreation, Indiana University–Bloomington*

Managers do things right; leaders do the right things.

Warren Bennis

One of the more important functions of the administrator of a department, school, or college is to develop and manage a solid fiscal base to support the programs and activities of the unit. It takes a combination of state, federal, private, and tuition funds to accomplish this task. Balancing these sources of revenue in order to provide resources for faculty productivity and student success is a necessary skill in modern administrative leadership. Too often, though, administrators become bound to the financial and budgetary aspects of the operation, and they are unable to exert imaginative and creative leadership over faculty, students, and programs. The skill of developing the financial base must be part of a combination of important functions discussed elsewhere in this book, including vision, planning, academic leadership, personnel administration, student services, and a myriad of other administrative duties.

In analyzing the approximate amount of time devoted to various administrative functions, it has been this writer's experience that almost half of one's time is spent on external duties such as alumni activities, professional activities, fundraising, and meetings with policy- and decision-makers on campus and in public office. The other half is spent on personnel issues, budgetary administration, program administration, and a host of routine administrative duties. All of the activities required to secure and administer the financial affairs of the unit take up a significant amount of the administrator's time and effort.

Ideally, programs should drive the financial and budgetary aspects of a unit instead of the other way around. Subsequently, it is extremely important to develop a strong vision and mission for the department, school, or college and to engage in continuous strategic planning to achieve the mission. A key part of the strategic function is the development of a financially stable revenue base and a meaningful and useful expenditure budget.

Another extremely important factor is the participation of other administrators in the unit (e.g., associate deans, department chairs, assistant chairs, budget officers). In addition, key faculty advisory committees and the faculty in general should have some involvement in the financial plan. The dean or department chair must ultimately manage the process, but participation by all individuals involved will provide significant dividends as the program moves forward. There are at least three levels in which administrative colleagues and faculty members may be involved in the planning process: the informational level, the consultative level, and the participative level. Whenever possible, the planning process should be decentralized to reflect a "bottom-up" as opposed to a "top-down" approach to governance (Chabotar, 1995, pp. 21-22). The desires and aspirations of the faculty should be included in the development of the financial plan. This process of involvement is absolutely necessary, not only because of the collegial nature of the decision-making process in the university, but also because it is nearly impossible for the dean or chair to know all of the forces that should come into play in such a plan. There are several mechanisms commonly used by deans and chairs to consult with colleagues before decisions are made about priorities and financial allocations related to the resource plan. However, most any such mechanism that involves a consultative and participative process will add strength to final decisions. In most cases, the chair or the dean must make the final decisions, but such judgments should be based on maximum input (Tucker & Bryan, 1991, pp. 58-60.)

The budget manager is responsible for putting together both the revenue and expenditure sides of the budget for the administrative unit. These include:

Revenue Sources

State allocation
Tuition and fees
Sponsored research
Endowment support
Gifts and grants
Investment incomes
Auxiliary enterprises

Expenditures

Instruction
Administrative departments
Capital equipment
Debt service
Reserve requirements
Auxiliary enterprises
Contingency

The first step in preparing a budget is to determine what the expected revenues will be for the next year (Lenington, 1996, p. 117). The process of preparing the expenditure budget will be discussed in chapter 18.

The categories listed above may be viewed from several perspectives by different stakeholders in the higher-education arena. They should be treated as broad categories by most deans and chairs in health, physical education, recreation, and dance (HPERD). There are considerable differences in the approaches to these sources of revenue between public and private institutions as well as between research-oriented and teaching-oriented institutions.

One of the primary sources of funds for public institutions is the allocation from the state legislature. This is often a standard amount, with incremental increases or decreases that are usually based on historical data and the current financial situation in the state. In some states, the allocation is formula-driven and based on enrollment and other factors at individual institutions. Once an institution receives these funds, they are internally allocated to its various units. Again, this internal allocation may be based on historical increments or on a formula basis. In some cases, colleges, schools, or departments may receive funds based on program expansion and new initiatives.

A second major source of revenue comes in the form of tuition and fees. While this source is a significant amount at public institutions, it constitutes an even larger proportion of the budget income at private schools. Differential tuition rates for in-state and out-of-state students exist in many public institutions, and these rates will vary depending on the mix of in-state and out-of-state students on campus. There is also income from a variety of miscellaneous fees (e.g., course fees, laboratory fees, student activity fees). This is particularly evident in HPERD units, given their preponderance of intramural and recreational sport programs that require lab fees, equipment fees, and other activity-related fees. Fees may also exist for services such as fitness and wellness programs, facility rentals, and lockers. In some cases, sales income may be generated from items such as disposable equipment, uniforms, logo items, and concessions.

Grants and contracts are another source of revenue, particularly for large research institutions (although they are becoming an increasingly important source for all institution types). Sponsored research dollars made available by corporations, foundations, and state and federal government agencies fund many major projects in institutions throughout the country. Funded projects often take the form of a contract for a particular service to be rendered such as comprehensive planning or the delivery of training programs or instructional units. These grants and contracts often provide for indirect or overhead administrative costs associated with the projects. The amount of indirect or overhead compensation provided will vary from agency to agency; this factor is quite significant, since these expenses can represent 50 percent or more of the total project cost. It is not uncommon, however, for state agencies to withhold such revenue from public institutions based on the contention that the state is already paying for these costs through its legislative appropriation. Indirect and overhead administrative costs are intended to pay for items such as staff support, equipment, building space, and administrative effort.

In general, grants and contracts have become an increasingly important part of the funding base for many institutions. As a result, it is not uncommon for many institutions to require that senior faculty members in particular secure sufficient amounts of grant and contract funding to cover

Sources of Revenue

their respective salaries. HPERD units have several sources of grant and contract possibilities. These include the National Institutes of Health, U.S. Department of Education, National Endowment for the Arts, National Park Service, and various other agencies across the country. Grants from these organizations are usually for research or training activities.

A final broad category of revenue consists of gifts, endowments, and other private support. This has long been a significant source of revenue for private institutions. In recent years, this source of funding has become increasingly prevalent at public institutions as well, and it is absolutely essential to the maintenance of high-quality programs at both types of institutions. Virtually all senior-level administrators, and some faculty, are involved in fundraising, development, and institutional advancement. These functions will be discussed in detail in later chapters. Most institutions have established foundations or some other legal structures that provide for tax-deductible gifts that can be used to support specific programs or pre-established endowments. Contributions can be made in the form of cash gifts or deferred requests, and they are usually designated for specific activities. Endowed chairs and endowed professorships have been very common in other disciplines for many years, but HPERD units have only recently placed an emphasis on this revenue source. Several universities have experienced great success in securing endowments for chairs and professorships. The income from the investment on the endowments supports the work of particular professors, specific student scholarships, or other similar activities. Corporate support and partnerships also provide support for program activities, but these may require advertisements or other services in return. Equipment manufacturers, particularly shoe companies and laboratory-equipment companies, have been particularly active participants in such relationships. Gifts are often made for equipment or buildings that usually involve naming opportunities or some other form of recognition for the organization (e.g., named scholarships, endowed professorships and chairs).

Change in Revenue Amounts

The proportion of the total revenue of an institution represented by each of the sources above varies dramatically, depending on the type of institution (particularly on whether it is public or private). The most obvious variation is that private institutions receive little or no funds from their state and, therefore, charge proportionately higher tuition and fees. Private institutions also depend more heavily on endowment funding for support. Among public institutions, research-oriented universities command significantly more funding from grants and contracts than teaching-oriented institutions. It is difficult, if not impossible, to classify institutions in discreet categories, since rules and functions within higher education continue to blend together, regardless of institution type. However, it is still useful to provide some broad guidelines that address the proportional distribution of income.

When analyzing all types of public institutions, the percentages of various revenue sources average out as follows: state government, 35 percent; tuition, 20 percent; grants and contracts, 15 percent; sales and services, 20 percent; gifts and endowments, 5 percent; and other sources, 5 percent. At private institutions, the approximate breakdown is: tuition and fees, 45 percent; grants and contracts, 20 percent; gifts and endowments, 10 percent; sales and services, 20 percent; and other sources, 5 percent (Callan &

Finney, 1997, p. 32). At several large public research institutions, the percentage of state appropriation support has dwindled to as low as 10 percent of the total budget. This has resulted in an increase in tuition, grants, contracts, gifts, endowments, and other sources of funds.

During the 1970s, tuition remained stable, or even declined, in public institutions across the United States, and remained relatively even with inflation at private institutions. However, during the last 20 years, tuition at both public and private institutions has increased substantially faster than inflation (St. John, 1994, p. 46). This trend is troubling to many who study the progress of higher education. It will be discussed more fully in a later section.

Institutional leaders must strive to maintain an appropriate balance in the sources of revenue that affect operating budgets. However, deans and department chairs in HPERD may have little control over these sources except in the categories of fees for services, grants, and contracts (which are credited directly to the unit, to be used for the purpose specified in the original agreement). As a result, securing additional grants and contracts will certainly enhance the revenue base within the unit. In some institutions, the indirect or overhead funds are held by the central administration, and in other institutions, at least a portion of these funds are returned to the unit securing the grant. Otherwise, central administration usually allocates funds to the college, school, or department. As a result, the unit administrator may not know the source or quantity of most of these funds.

Budgeting Systems

The institutional budgeting process is more fully addressed in another chapter. However, it is appropriate to offer some brief comments about budgeting systems here due to the increased trend of allowing internal units to exert more control over their sources of funds. There are several approaches to budgeting, and each approach is distinctive in its emphasis on different kinds of information. Incremental budgeting focuses primarily on increases or decreases to the base budget that has existed in previous years. Planning, programming, and budgeting systems (PPBS) weigh the costs and benefits of programs and activities in a unit and focus on the substance of these programs. Zero-based budgeting examines all programs and activities during each budget cycle and assesses their relative merits. Performance budgeting focuses on measures of programs or activity performance outcomes and places a value on these through the budget. Formula budgeting is concerned mainly with "fair share" distribution sources among programs as determined by some quantitative measures. Cost-centered budgeting or responsibility-centered budgeting focuses on the relative ability of a unit to be self-supporting (Meisinger, 1994, p. 171).

The latter system of responsibility-centered management represents an attempt to decentralize the financial operations of the university in order to place incentives at the lowest reasonable levels of accountability. In its simplest form, this system returns all income generated by the responsibility center—usually a school or college—to the unit represented by that center. In addition to a pre-determined allocation from the state (in the case of public institutions), the responsibility-center unit also receives all of the tuition and fees earned through credit hours generated from registrations in its classes, indirect or overhead funds generated from its grants and contracts, and any other income it earns. The responsibility center is then assessed fees or taxes based on sophisticated algorithms that pay for central university costs such as library, registrar, financial aid, building space, central administration, and so forth. This system provides a basis for the unit to receive all income generated from the tuition of students taught in its classes along with other fees and indirect costs. In other words, units that teach more students and generate more grant income receive everything that they have earned. Obviously, this is an incentive system that places the responsibility for income and cost on the responsibility center and at the lowest level possible within the university. The responsibility-center administrators are expected to manage the resources at their disposal in order to maximize their performance (Whalen, 1991). This system does, in fact, give responsibility-center administrators a great deal of discretion and control over income generation. Since the responsibility center is usually at the school or college level, the dean is normally in a position to exercise significant authority in fiscal decision-making. However, some responsibility centers transfer these operating principles to the department level, which enables individual department chairs to wield important discretion. Several large public and private universities are now experimenting with various forms of responsibility-centered management.

Qualitative Issues

Every successful administrator is concerned with maintaining high-quality programs, and this task is not always easy to evaluate. The process of building a stable financial base to support high-quality programs is begun by setting priorities for the division, mission, and strategic plan of the unit. How does a dean or chair set these priorities? In general, this must be done after a great deal of consultation with department chairs or program leaders and faculty. The key word here is "consultation." Consultation does not mean "taking votes," because vote-taking cannot realistically be accomplished in a setting as large as a school or college. Ultimately, one individual must take responsibility for these decisions, usually the dean or the chair. Decision-making is not always easy, but it is a part of the role of a unit administrator. It is not possible for a committee of department chairs or program leaders to decide which one or two of their respective departments or programs should receive preferential treatment in the allocation of resources. Chairs and program leaders should have an opportunity to present an argument for fair and equitable treatment, and the dean or chair will ultimately evaluate that argument along with other considerations in order to make a fair decision. These considerations cover a broad range of topics, including: the strengths and weaknesses of the programs or department; the internal arrangements of the college, school, or department with other units in the institution; the needs of society, which may or may not be the same as marketplace consideration; the opportunities provided to students within the department or program; and the desires and aspirations of the faculty. Not all programs can be evaluated as "highest priority," and not all faculty aspirations can be fulfilled. However, the consultative process ensures that the dean or chair is receiving the best input for making good decisions relative to the allocation of resources (Tucker & Bryan, 1991).

Resource allocation must necessarily address faculty quality and productivity. There are few issues in higher education that receive more attention—but less valid measurement—than faculty productivity. The reason is that faculty members perform so many different roles and functions that it is hard to quantify and compare their activities. Who can measure the productivity of a creative mind? Is it possible to quantify in any meaningful way the effectiveness of a great teacher? What is the value of a piece of research? How much is a "full load"? These and other questions abound, but they must be addressed by every dean or department chair if the academic unit is to be effective. Space does not permit a full discussion of these issues here, but the answers to these and other questions about productivity and workload must ultimately be found by initiating and maintaining a continuing dialogue with faculty about this matter (Tierney, 1999). Most faculty want to be productive, and this can usually be achieved through guidance, consultation, and a continuing evaluation process. Salary increases will usually not motivate faculty members to be more productive. This fact stems from the intrinsic values that characterize faculty members with respect to their place in the department and their desire to contribute to the mission of the university.

Accountability and cost containment have received a great deal of attention in higher education in recent years. Deans and department chairs have an increased responsibility to manage their programs in a way that ensures efficient use of existing and scarce resources. There are, of course, uncontrollable costs in any operation. However, there are also more proactive opportunities for deans and chairs to control expenses than what might first be perceived. For example, the HPERD administrator must look at issues such as the design of a focused curriculum in physical education, the number of courses in the recreation and parks program, the number and size of sections taught in health, the elimination of predictably unproductive programs and courses in the basic instruction program, the reduction of student attrition, the use of new technologies, faculty workload considerations, and the close monitoring of the copy machine and travel budget (Simpson, 1991). While it may not be obvious at first, it is more cost-effective to employ the very best, most highly qualified faculty possible. The most highly qualified faculty are usually more expensive, but they are usually the most productive as well. In the long run, they will cost less than lower-salaried faculty with fewer qualifications and abilities.

Trends in Funding Higher Education

Clearly, society's expectations of higher education, along with the public's willingness to pay for it, are changing dramatically. Virtually all authorities in higher education agree that certain financial trends will undoubtedly shape the future of all institutions. While certain trends will affect different disciplines in different ways, all of the trends will have an impact on deans and chairs in HPERD.

One such trend is the dramatic decline in state funding for public institutions during the last several years. As a result of leaner state budgets, state policy-makers and legislators have been forced to make difficult spending decisions and policy choices. The proportion of state budget allocations earmarked for higher education has been in decline since 1997; states have redirected state funds to other need areas such as primary and secondary education, Medicare, transportation, and corrections. The public is no longer completely confident that institutions of higher education are using their funds efficiently; thus there may be a belief that universities can in fact operate with smaller budgets. At the federal level, some of these same factors are at work. Except for health-related issues, there is a much more uncertain future regarding federal funding for university-based research. This is likely to have a major impact on the larger research universities (Hossler, 1997; Zusman, 1999).

With comparatively less state funding and federal research dollars, institutions will be forced to look to other sources of income such as increased tuition and fees, more grants and contracts from sources other than the federal government, and more contributions from private sources. Deans and chairs in HPERD have little control over some of these factors. Grants, contracts, fees for services, and private contributions are likely to offer the most promise to administrators as they strive to support programs in these fields in the future.

Summary

Today's financial climate forces the administrator to be very creative in securing funds and managing them for various programs. It is extremely important that administrators do not become obsessed with the difficulties of supporting programs; they must remain focused on the positive contributions that these programs make to the quality of life in modern society. After more than 30 years as a dean or chair, this writer continues to be extremely optimistic about the future of the HPERD fields. Our society has undergone a fundamental change in its perception of fitness, sport, leisure, and safe and healthful living. There is simply no evidence to suggest that these perceptions will go away any time soon. Partly as a result, it will be necessary to become more aggressive and creative in the procurement of funds. After many years in administration, I do not have much naiveté left. However, I continue to believe that there is funding out there for every good program, whether it is dedicated to service, instruction, or research. When resources are tight, it is necessary to set priorities, insist on high-quality programs, expect accountability, and work on cost-containment. It may take hard work and some imagination, but funding opportunities for such programs do exist; there is almost always a source of support for high-quality activities in HPERD.

The successful administrator must take a "can do" approach to obtaining funds for good programs. It is usually a bad idea to say "no" to any request from faculty or staff for funding a new idea. Funds might not always be available, but the first response should be, "Let's see if there is a way that this can be done." The dean or chair should give faculty members an opportunity to assist in the exploration of revenue sources to support these ideas. It is always amazing to see the results when several good minds are focused on this endeavor. In the event that funds simply cannot be found, faculty members will walk away with the feeling that every effort was made and that they have been supported. Again, though, there is usually a way to fund worthwhile projects and programs.

About the Author

Tony A. Mobley is dean of, and a professor in, the School of Health, Physical Education, and Recreation at Indiana University–Bloomington. He has been a dean or department chair for more than 30 years at three different universities.

References

Callan, P. M., & Finney, J. E. (1997). *Public and private financing of higher education: Shaping public policy for the future.* Phoenix, AZ: Oryx.

Chabotar, K. J. (1995). Managing participative budgeting in higher education. *Change,* September/October, 21-22.

Hossler, D. (1997). State funding for higher education: The Sisyphean task. *Journal of Higher Education, 68*(2), 160-190.

Lenington, R. L. (1996). *Managing higher education as a business.* Phoenix, AZ: Oryx.

Meisinger, R. J. (1994). *College and university budgeting: An introduction for faculty and academic administrators.* Washington, DC: National Association of College and University Business Officers.

St. John, E. P. (1994). *Prices, productivity, and investment: Assessing financial strategies in higher education.* Washington, DC: George Washington University.

Simpson, W. B. (1991). *Cost containment for higher education: Strategies for public policy and institutional administration,* Westport, CT: Praeger.

Tierney, W. G. (1999). *Building the responsive campus: Creating high performance colleges and universities.* Thousand Oaks, CA: Sage.

Tucker, A., & Bryan, R. (1991). *The academic dean: Dove, dragon, and diplomat.* New York: American Council on Education.

Whalen, E. L. (1991). *Responsibility-centered* budgeting: *An approach to decentralized management for institutions of higher education.* Bloomington, IN: Indiana University Press.

Zusman, A. (1999). *Issues facing higher education in the 21st century.* Baltimore: Johns Hopkins University Press.

16 Encouraging Faculty to Obtain Grants

Dana D. Brooks, *Professor and Dean, School of Physical Education, West Virginia University*

Seek council, listen and reflect before you make a decision.

⊶ Dana D. Brooks

The Kellogg Commission on the Future of State and Land-Grant Universities (1997, 1998, 1999a,b) and the Boyer Commission on Educating Undergraduates in the Research University (1998) challenged higher-education administrators to reassess their commitment to promoting academic excellence throughout their institutions. Canvassing the current status of higher education in America, the Kellogg Commission (1998, 1999a) offered the following general recommendations for colleges and universities that wish to strengthen their values and educational missions: such institutions should (1) become student-centered learning communities, (2) provide an environment for students to engage in research, (3) value student diversity, (4) maintain fiscal responsibility, (5) encourage interdisciplinary scholarship and research, and (6) foster lifelong learning. These recommendations are interwoven with the following propositions: (1) institutions must increase research/scholarship activities in all areas (including teaching and service), and (2) the preservation of knowledge is important to our culture and remains an important mission within American higher education. Yet there are many internal and external forces (political, economic, social) impacting the future of higher education and of health, physical education, recreation, and dance (HPERD) programs.

Fiscal realities will continue to have a major impact on higher-education reform. As Gardner (1999) asserted, "The funding of public higher education nearly everywhere in the U.S. ebbs and flows with the times" (p. 21). Ruppert (1996) reminded us that while the amount of funding granted to public universities has grown steadily, the actual percentage of state general-revenue budgets spent on higher education witnessed a downturn from 1990-95. As a result of these new fiscal

153

realities, many higher-education administrators are now adopting a business approach to revenue.

Like it or not, many colleges and universities today are "public assisted" rather than "public supported" (Edginton, Davis, & Hensley, 1994, p. 53). In an attempt to offset reduced state funding for academic programs and spiraling internal costs, many institutions are increasing student enrollment, tuition, and fees and relying more on private and alumni support. In addition, deans and chairs are asking (and in some cases demanding) that faculty write and submit research grants and contracts for possible external funding. Within academia, the term "contract" usually refers to "a funding mechanism used to secure a product according to a funding source's organizationally determined specifications" (Ries & Leukefeld, 1995, p. 56). In contrast, grants are usually financial awards provided to support research and other scholarly activities. Unfortunately, many faculty members do not have the expertise to successfully negotiate the grants and contracts gauntlet.

When I began my academic career as an assistant professor, I was motivated to write and submit grant proposals to support my research agenda in the area of sport sociology. Yet I soon realized that my formal education had not prepared me for the complexities of this process. When preparing my grant proposals, I began to interact with the university's Office of Sponsored Programs, my dean's office budget staff, and various outside funding agencies (federal, state, and private). During these interactions, I was expected to have some knowledge about the duties of the principal investigator, the indirect cost of facilities and administration, the current fringe-benefit rates negotiated between the institution and the U.S. Department of Health and Human Services, intellectual property (including patents, copyrights, and trademarks), acceptable budget development, and how to identify potential funding agencies. Several times, I became very frustrated with this process, which proved to be very labor-intensive, with little or no possibility of reward (i.e., grant not funded, and no credit given for developing the proposal as part of my research expectations for promotion and tenure). The purpose of this chapter, based on my personal experience and the existing literature, is twofold: (1) to identify institutional and personal barriers that faculty members and administrators must eliminate if they are going to achieve any measure of success in the grants/contracts marketplace, and (2) to discuss strategies for enhancing the possibility of receiving external funding to support teaching, research, and service activities.

Barriers to Developing Grant and Contract Proposals

The traditional definition of scholarship must change to reflect a new set of faculty expectations and institutional and societal needs (Scott & Awbrey, 1993). For example, many colleges and universities now consider the writing and submitting of grant proposals as a "scholarly" activity. Several scholars and administrators have long recognized the value and significance of encouraging HPERD faculty to pursue grants and contracts. As Aufsesser and Mechikoff (1984) asserted, if we are going "to maintain the quality of current programs and to expand or enhance future projects, we must compete for funds from the corporate sector" (p. 69). Today, young scholars hired at research, doctoral, comprehensive, or undergraduate institutions are expected to write and submit grants and contracts to meet promotion and tenure guidelines. Highlighting this point,

Ries and Leukefeld (1995) wrote, "Professionals are expected to have funded research or evaluation projects early in their careers….[Academics] who did not consider research (much less externally funded research) important to their professional progress now find it to be an integral part of their advancement and promotion" (p. 11).

Why are universities placing so much emphasis on writing, submitting, and receiving external funding? The answer is simple: grants and contracts constitute a multi-billion-dollar-per-year industry (Miner & Griffith, 1993). A portion of the facilities and administration rates (i.e., compensation provided by funding agencies to support institutional expenses, construction and maintenance of facilities, etc.) may be used to support an institution's mission. On a more practical level, "The largest percentage of funds generated by research grants goes to pay salaries of graduate students, research professionals, and principal investigators. The next largest fraction is spent on developing research facilities" (Research Task Force White Pages: Educational Value of Research, 1996, p. 5). In some situations, these funds also support library acquisitions.

Furthermore, institutions receive prestige, rewards, and visibility based on the number of external grants secured by their faculty. According to Boyer and Cockriel (1998), "Research Universities judge themselves— and are judged by others—based on research productivity and the dollar amount [of] acquired grants" (p. 61). Similarly, the Boyer Commission (1998) reported that "the standing of a university is measured by the research productivity of its faculty: the place of a department within the university is determined by whether its members garner more or fewer research dollars" (p. 7). Writing and receiving grants and contracts also enhances individual faculty members' professional reputations (Boyer & Cockriel, 1998).

The literature clearly suggests that the success rate for obtaining grants and contracts is tied to a nurturing and supportive campus community. Deans and chairs have a responsibility to create a campus environment and infrastructure that supports and values all forms of research and scholarship, including grant activity. Monahan (1993) eloquently described the risks, rewards, and faculty expectations associated with developing grant proposals: "Faculty further want their institutions to demonstrate the value placed on grants as a form of scholarly activity by providing greater recognition of their work, not only in college and other publications but also in the tenure and promotion decision process" (p. 22).

In an effort to ascertain impediments to faculty grant-writing, Monahan (1993) surveyed the faculty of eight state colleges in New Jersey. Initially, the researcher identified a list of potential obstacles to grant development:

- Heavy teaching load
- Heavy student-advising load
- Committee assignments
- Departmental administration's lack of training in writing and seeking grants
- No colleagues with whom to work
- Lack of knowledge about budgeting.

Removing Obstacles and Sharing Responsibility

The data revealed that a large percentage of the faculty at these colleges did not engage in grant-related activities because they were not seeking promotion or tenure. In addition, they reported that teaching and advising loads prevented them from engaging in such activities (though it must be noted that undergraduate education was the primary mission of the eight institutions in this study).

Similarly, Boyer and Cockriel (1998) surveyed faculty in the College of Education at the University of Missouri–Columbia to determine what barriers, if any, were keeping faculty from developing grant proposals. They found that lack of training and knowledge, coupled with the general difficulty of locating funding sources, were significant disincentives to developing grant proposals. These findings were especially true for non-tenured faculty.

HPERD faculty members face similar problems in their quest for external funding. Unfortunately, very few doctorate-granting programs in these fields require students to develop grant and contract proposals as an integral part of their studies.

Breaking down the barriers to successful grants and contracts development must begin with the institution's commitment to valuing these and other forms of externally sponsored scholarship. Building an environment that fosters the acquisition of grants and contracts is a joint responsibility of faculty and administrators. The university must have the infrastructure (at the college and department level) to support grants and contracts, and faculty must be motivated to develop proposals and rewarded for doing so.

Based on best practices described in the literature, it is evident that administrators must be willing to provide flexibility and balance in teaching, research, and service. Boyer (1990) challenged higher education to re-examine faculty priorities and move away from the traditional debate of teaching versus research when considering faculty rewards. Similarly, the Kellogg Commission (1998) strongly encouraged a change in the faculty reward system, recommending that the correlations between good undergraduate teaching and good research (including sponsored research) be recognized in promotion and tenure decisions. Clearly, faculty promotion and tenure guidelines must articulate the institutional and departmental expectations for faculty grant-writing and acquisition. Today, writing, submitting, and receiving external research grants is a reasonable expectation for faculty members seeking promotion or tenure, particularly for faculty at doctoral and research institutions. It is also important to remember that the publication of grant- or contract-funded research findings in high-quality, peer-reviewed journals remains a high priority at most institutions, especially for faculty seeking promotion and tenure. The Carnegie Foundation for the Advancement of Teaching (1989) has noted that faculty from all types of institutions tend to agree that it is difficult for a person to be tenured and promoted if he/she does not publish on a regular basis.

Infrastructure Support: University Level

New faculty orientation. It is imperative for institutions to conduct orientation sessions for new faculty (usually before the first week of classes). During such sessions, it is important to highlight services provided by the institution's office of sponsored programs. Topics covered during the orientation sessions should include:

- Duties and responsibilities of the office of sponsored programs
- Overview of the institution's grants and contracts submission procedures

- Grant submission deadlines
- Required approval signatures on all grants submitted
- Names of institutional representatives
- Compliance issues (e.g., human or animal subjects)
- Oversight (e.g., how an award from a sponsor is processed)
- Intellectual property
- Proprietary material.

Office of sponsored programs and grant accountability. The preliminary step in writing and submitting grants and contracts is contacting key individuals in the institution's office of sponsored programs. This office can help faculty locate potential funding sources, develop and clarify the formal proposal, develop a proposed budget and check it for accuracy, and, finally, submit the proposal to the appropriate funding agency on behalf of the institution. Once the grant or contract is received, this office works closely with the central administration budget office and the appropriate dean's office to ensure that grant funds are transferred to the correct funding accounts. It is critical that the office of sponsored programs have staff and other resources available to help faculty with fiscal reports, audit review, interim reports, subsequent contracts, budget management, and compliance with all agency guidelines.

University-allocated seed money to support faculty research. Numerous universities have established faculty research grant programs to stimulate research activities. For example, Memphis State University (MSU) funded a total of approximately $600,000 in faculty awards from 1985 to 1991. DeHart's (1993) assessment of the MSU Faculty Research Incentive Program highlighted the grant recipients' belief that internal grants had a positive impact on their ability to obtain external research grants.

The ultimate success of a grant or contract is tied to the level of departmental support for it. Academic departments must have technical, financial, and personnel resources readily available to help faculty complete grants and contracts.

Budget-development and management support. Clearly, research-grant budgets represent only an estimate of anticipated costs. Yet, for the novice faculty member, developing such a budget can be a challenge. Usually, budgets for grants and contracts include personnel costs (e.g., salaries, wages, fringe benefits) and non-personnel cost (e.g., travel, supplies, equipment). In many situations, agency and university policies, procedures, and guidelines dictate how budgets are developed and administered.

Department, school, or college budget office managers should work very closely with faculty members as they prepare grants and contracts for submission. Once a grant or contract is awarded, local budget officers should provide the faculty member with regular budget summary reports. It is an important to remember that academic deans serve as the chief fiscal officers for all grants and contracts awarded to faculty assigned to their academic unit. Technically, grants and contracts are awarded to institutions, not to individual faculty members. Faculty members serve as principal investigators working on behalf of the institution. Thus, it is imperative that deans (or their designees) closely monitor all grant and contract activities. In addition, deans should be familiar with all federal, state, and institutional regulations pertinent to any grant or contract.

Infrastructure Support: College/ Department Level

Financial support. Establishing start-up funds at the local level can serve as an incentive for faculty to develop grant and contract proposals. One example of a successful incentive program is the use of "seed money" awards. Departments or colleges can establish these financial awards to help junior faculty members with their research. The purpose of this initiative is to make funding available (on a competitive basis), thus providing opportunities for professional growth and future acquisition of external grants. "seed money" grants can be used to conduct pilot research, pay human subjects, fund travel for data collection, or purchase lab and computer equipment.

Another good incentive program for faculty is an "External Funding Incentive Salary Plan." Such programs can motivate faculty to write and procure external grants and contracts. It is important to note that such incentive programs must first be approved by the office of the provost and the office of sponsored programs. Below are sample guidelines for an external funding incentive salary program (note that these guidelines refer to proportional—rather than fixed—rates for faculty compensation):

- Faculty members may earn up to 20 percent of their base salary.
- Any faculty member receiving unpaid release time for grant-related activity has access to 75 percent of the grant funds (provided that this proportion does not exceed 20 percent of his or her normal base salary).
- The faculty member's department will receive 15 percent of the funds. In addition, the department will receive any "principal investigator" funds above 20 percent of the faculty member's base salary.
- The dean's office will receive 10 percent of the funds. Any funds received by the dean's office are generally reallocated as seed money to support additional faculty research projects.

A "Personnel and Professional Network Support System" can also help faculty write and submit grants and contracts. In an attempt to establish various support structures, deans and chairs are encouraged to:

- Establish a formal networking system that pairs faculty members who have experience in obtaining grants and contracts with novice faculty members. These mentors should read proposals, help identify funding sources, assist with research design and data analysis, guide budget preparation, and so forth.
- Conduct seminars on "in-house" grants and contracts. The purpose of such seminars is to link faculty members with existing internal sources for grants and contracts. Deans, office budget managers, and guest speakers from the office of sponsored programs, the provost's office, and the human subjects research approval committee should all be invited to meet with faculty on a regular basis.

Departments should also provide funding, when necessary, for faculty to attend seminars on grants and contracts both within and outside the university. Such seminars can enhance faculty members' knowledge base and expand their support network for grants and contracts. Furthermore, the dean's office should compile and maintain a list of potential HPERD funding agencies. *The Annual Register of Grant Support: A Directory of Funding Sources* (1998) is an excellent resource for faculty attempting to identify potential funding sources. For example, the following entries are included in this resource:

◆ **Amateur Athletic Foundation of Los Angeles**
2141 West Adams Boulevard
Los Angeles, CA 90018
213-730-9600
FAX: 213-730-9637

Areas of Interest: Youth sports
Types: Capital Grants: challenge/matching grants; project/program grants. Field of physical activity.
Purpose: To promote and enhance youth sports opportunities in Southern California.

◆ **American Kinesiotherapy Association, Inc.**
P.O. Box 5188
Vancouver, WA 98668-5188
800-296-AKTA

Areas of Interest: Kinesiotherapy, including adapted physical education
Types: Scholarships, awards for students in AKTA-accredited kinesiotherapy programs.
Purpose: Recognition of academic excellence and career planning through funding for educational needs.

◆ **American Health Assistance Foundation**
15825 S. Shady Grove Road
Suite 140
Rockville, MD 20850
301-948-3244
FAX: 301-258-9454

Areas of Interest: Stroke and cardiovascular disease
Types: Research Grants. Awards for research on the causes and potential treatments of stroke and cardiovascular disease.
Purpose: To assist young investigators at the level of Assistant Professor or equivalent who are starting a research program.

◆ **New Jersey State Council on the Arts**
20 West State Street, 3rd Floor
Trenton, NJ 08625
609-292-6130
FAX: 609-989-1440

Areas of Interest: Dance, music, mime, opera, etc.
Types: Block grants, fellowships, general operating grants, residencies

◆ **New York State Council on the Arts**
915 Broadway
New York, NY 10010
212-387-7000
FAX: 212-387-7164

Areas of Interest: Funding of the arts in the state of New York
Types: Capital Grants: modeling grants, residencies

From The Annual Register Of Grant Support: A Directory of Funding Sources (1998)

The Foundation Directory (Falkenstein & Jacobs, 1999) is another excellent resource for faculty seeking grants and contracts. It identified 2,181 grant-allocating foundations in 1999, and it is edited and updated annually.

Finally, do not forget to use the World Wide Web to find potential funding from federal and state agencies or private foundations. Specifically, SPIN (a web-based product offered by InfoEd International; see http://australia.infoed.org/) provides world-wide searches for funding opportunities, and the GENIUS and SMARTS systems (also from InfoEd) list funding opportunities on a daily basis.

Summary

Current trends in higher education suggest that schools, colleges, and departments of kinesiology, physical education, and health will need to rely more on grants and contracts to support faculty research agendas and institutional missions. Yet few researchers in the fields of HPERD and sport studies have systematically investigated barriers and incentives to successful procurement of grants and contracts. Nonetheless, many articles published since the 1970s have indicated that lack of time, lack of technical knowledge (e.g., about identifying funding sources and budgeting), lack of administrative support, and lack of rewards (e.g., promotion, tenure, public recognition) are all significant barriers to faculty members' success in obtaining such funding (Monahan, 1993). Administrative incentives to redress these barriers include: faculty release time to develop grant proposals; establishment of an infrastructure that supports all phases of the grant and contract submission process; and administrative support and rewards for faculty who receive grants and contracts.

About the Author

Dana D. Brooks is a professor in, and the dean of, the School of Physical Education at West Virginia University. He has been involved in higher education for 11 years.

References

Annual register of grant support: A directory of funding sources (31st ed.). (1998). New Providence, NJ: R.R. Bowker.

Aufsesser, P. M., & Mechikoff, R. (1984). Grantsmanship and external funding: The paper chase. *Journal of Physical Education, Recreation & Dance, 55*(6), 69, 76.

Boyer, E. L. (1990). *Scholarship reconsidered: Priorities of the professoriate.* Lawrenceville, NJ: Princeton University Press.

Boyer, P., & Cockriel, I. (1998). Factors influencing grant writing: Perceptions of tenured and non-tenured faculty. *SRA Journal, 29*(3-4), 61-68.

Boyer Commission on Educating Undergraduates in the Research University. (1998). *Reinventing undergraduate education: A blueprint for America's research universities* [On-line]. Available: http://notes.cc.sunysb.edu/Pres/boyer.nsf

Carnegie Foundation for the Advancement of Teaching. (1989). *The conditions of the professionals: Attitudes and trends.* Princeton, NJ: Princeton University Press.

DeHart, V. J. (1993). Internal faculty research grants program: An effective component of research programs. *SRA Journal, 24*(4), 5-8.

Edginton, C. R., Thomas, M. D., & Hensley, L. D. (1994). Trends in higher education: Implications for health, physical education, and leisure studies. *Journal of Physical Education, Recreation and Dance, 65*(7), 51-57.

Falkenstein, J. A., & Jacobs, D. G. (Eds.). (1999). *The foundation directory.* New York: The Foundation Center.

Gardner, D. P. (1999). Meeting the challenges of the new millennium: The university's role. In W. Z. Hirsch & L. E. Weber (Eds.), *Challenges facing higher education at the millennium* (pp. 18-25). Phoenix, AZ: Oryx.

Kellogg Commission on the Future of State and Land-Grant Universities. (1997). *Returning to our roots: The student experience.* Washington, DC: National Association of State Universities and Land-Grant Colleges.

Kellogg Commission on the Future of State and Land-Grant Universities. (1998). *Returning to our roots: Student access.* Washington, DC: National Association of State Universities and Land-Grant Colleges.

Kellogg Commission on the Future of State and Land-Grant Universities. (1999a). *Returning to our roots: The engaged institution.* Washington, DC: National Association of State Universities and Land-Grant Colleges.

Kellogg Commission on the Future of State and Land-Grant Universities. (1999b). *Returning to our roots: A learning society.* Washington, DC: National Association of State Universities and Land-Grant Colleges.

Miner, L. E., & Griffith, J. (1993). *Proposal planning and writing.* Phoenix, AZ: Oryx.

Monahan, T. C. (1993). Barriers and inducements to grant-related activity by New Jersey State College faculty. *Journal of the Society of Research Administrators, 25*(4), 9-25.

Research task force white pages: Educational value of research. (1996, April 30). Morgantown, WV: West Virginia University.

Ries, J. B., & Leukefeld, C. G. (1995). *Applying for research funding: Getting started and getting funded.* Thousand Oaks, CA: Sage.

Ruppert, S. (1996). *The politics of remedy: State legislative views on higher education.* Washington, DC: NEA National Center for Innovation and Office of Higher Education.

Scott, D. K., & Awbrey, S. M. (1993). Transforming scholarship. *Change, 25*(4), 38-43.

17 Fundraising: It Begins and Ends with Alumni

J. William Douglas, *Professor and Dean Emeritus, School of Physical Education, West Virginia University*

Successful administrators are those who expect success and diligently attempt to achieve it.

⊶ J. Wiliam Douglas

During the past decade, raising funds for public and private higher-education institutions has become increasingly important. *The Chronicle of Higher Education* and *Higher Education and National Affairs* are replete with articles describing program budget cuts, financial reversions, lost faculty positions, and even the development of plans for declaring financial emergency. Regrettably, program growth and enrichment has become more difficult as a result. Institutions must either rely solely on woefully insufficient appropriated budgets to support their programs or seek extramural financing from the private sector. While the thought of fundraising is distasteful to most faculty and many administrators in higher education, all appreciate the benefits derived from philanthropic gifts. Since the bulk of fundraising activity occurs at the program level (as opposed to the institution-wide development office), it is imperative that health, physical education, recreation, and dance (HPERD) personnel become involved. Unfortunately, most deans or chairs in this field have had no formal educational experience in such activity and are reluctant to retool. Others are convinced that most HPERD graduates either have insufficient wealth to make charitable gifts of any consequence or are more likely to bestow large gifts on intercollegiate athletic departments than on academic departments; thus, they feel that fundraising efforts would not be worthwhile. This latter attitude was held by my predecessor when I became a university dean in 1979.

Initially, I conducted annual fundraising campaigns without the benefit of having been professionally prepared, with an insufficient database of alumni, and with little financial success. Within five years, however, our

163

School of Physical Education had turned the corner and posted five-figure net receipts. By 1988, a $1 million capital campaign was successfully conducted by the school (as part of the university's goal of $150 million). This success was primarily due to the fact that fundraising had become an integral part of my job, even though this function was not initially a part of my position description. Today, fundraising is, presumably, an integral part of every dean's position. To be successful in this undertaking, it is necessary to become a student of fundraising; that is, to read publications of the Council for Advancement and Support of Education (CASE), to attend relevant workshops, and to understand the art and science of fundraising.

The "art" of fundraising involves developing a relationship between the fund-raiser and the prospective donor. This activity takes many forms, including periodic telephone calls, invitations to campus for homecoming celebrations, contacts through program newsletters, personal visitations in the home or office, and alumni receptions at professional meetings. The importance of alumni in fundraising is evidenced on the World Wide Web (e.g., a recent web search produced 626 references to alumni relations and fundraising) and in many of the articles printed in *Currents*, a publication of CASE. What might begin as a casual personal relationship between a dean, department chair, or faculty member and an alumnus of the institution may eventually result in a major gift transaction. It is imperative, therefore, that every graduate be treated as a prospective donor. While most major gifts will come as a result of intensive prospecting and cultivation, others will come without any advance notice, often during the settlement of an estate.

The "science" of fundraising requires that fund-raisers be able to match their organizational needs to the potential donor's wishes, and to execute the entire process, from prospecting to soliciting. This enables an annual campaign with a $100,000 goal or a five-year capital campaign with a $10 million goal to be realized. Successful fund-raisers will be knowledgeable of both the art and science of raising money during annual campaigns, planned giving, and capital campaigns. They will also understand that most donors begin by contributing a small annual gift and may progress (over an extended time frame) toward a larger, planned gift, perhaps as part of a capital campaign.

Annual Campaigns

Annual campaigns are conducted to generate funding necessary to provide the extras that make a program special. Such funding is rarely included in appropriated budgets. While fundraising events such as spaghetti dinners, magazine sales, elimination drawings, silent auctions, or golf outings have the potential to generate a large sum of money, the focus here will be on annual-campaign activities that, when combined, will generate $100,000 or more.

An annual campaign begins with an organizational plan and a case statement. The plan identifies who is to be solicited, how and when the solicitation will be made, and who will do the soliciting. The case statement describes why the campaign is being conducted and, more importantly, invites the prospective donor to participate. It also lists the fundraising activities that have been strategically planned throughout the year. Burdinski (2000) advanced the notion that strategic planning expresses the long-term vision of the campaign and is critical to its success. Fund-raisers must plan annual fund activities that are appropriate to the mission of the institution and a comprehensive campaign that will provide for a broad base of support. Examples of such activities are described below.

Telephone solicitation (i.e., a phone-athon) is a productive and cost-effective fundraising strategy, though many fund-raisers detest making telephone calls, especially "cold calls." Ideally, the calls would be made by the dean and/or those faculty who are likely to know or be known by the prospective donor. Unfortunately, deans do not have time for such calls, and faculty are, likewise, too busy and/or reluctant to assist. Thus, the calls are often made by students employed by the institution. If these students are to be successful, it is imperative that they be proficient in telling the fundraising "story" (which should be prepared in advance by program personnel).

Direct-mail campaigns are an inexpensive means of soliciting new donors and renewing the involvement of those who have not made a contribution for several years. The request should be written by a high-profile graduate who believes in the program. If possible, such requests should also be personalized with the prospective donor's name. Another form of mail contact is the *program newsletter*, whether disseminated by mail, e-mail, web site, or a combination of media. A fundraising article can be included in each issue, with a response form in which a cash gift can be made.

Class-reunion and challenge gifts are solicited by a prominent member of a particular graduating class who writes a letter to members of that class. To ensure the success of this activity, it is advisable to have a cadre of volunteers from the class who can make personal contacts. An "each one reach one" approach is an effective strategy.

Direct solicitation (i.e., one-on-one contact by the dean's development staff, the chair, or other campaign volunteers) is the most effective means of approaching a potential donor. It is also the most expensive, requires the greatest time commitment, and, due to geographical distance, may not be even be feasible. One alternative is to make contact at a homecoming reception or at state and national professional meetings. The size of the gift being sought will determine the appropriate solicitation strategy. Obviously, it is easier to obtain a large contribution when the solicitation is made in person and in private.

Lessons learned. To increase the success of an annual campaign, fund-raisers would be well-served by heeding the following lessons:

1. A strategic plan is imperative in procuring annual gifts.
2. An accurate and comprehensive Management Information System (MIS) of graduates, friends, corporations, and foundations must be created.
3. To the extent possible, direct solicitation should be used. A telephone call or mailing to a graduate 100 miles away is very inexpensive and may result in a $100 gift. A face-to-face meeting with this person may cost $100 and take several hours, but is likely to result in a gift of $1,000 or more.
4. At the end of the year, fundraising activity must be evaluated and the results reported to the program's constituents. This can be done using the program's newsletter.

5. Each gift should be appropriately recognized and rewarded (e.g., with a thank-you letter, a listing in a program newsletter, a plaque, or a framed picture of a noteworthy campus building, depending on the size of the gift).

Annual giving is an often used (and sometimes abused) means of raising money to increase operating revenue or to provide the little extras that are not available from the appropriated budget. Yet most institutions are looking for the "big money"—where one or a few planned gifts might exceed the sum of annual-campaign gifts.

Planned Giving

A planned gift is a voluntary gift of any kind, in any amount, given for any purpose (either current or deferred), that requires the assistance of a qualified professional to plan and manage (Sharpe, 1999, p. 1). Whereas an annual gift comes from one's disposable income, a planned gift comes from wealth (i.e., accumulated assets or possessions that will provide economic return now or later). Such "major" gifts (typically in excess of $25,000) complement annual gifts; they are the result of extensive cultivation and may not be available to beneficiaries for 10 to 15 years. Generally, they reduce the donor's estate, income, and/or capital-gains taxes. Examples of specific planned gifts often made to charitable institutions are described below.

Outright donations can include: cash or pledged cash installments; appreciated stocks; real property (e.g., land, homes, buildings); personal property (e.g., art, jewelry, and coin collections); and business inventory (including livestock).

Bequests are made through a will. This is a widely used means to transfer an asset from an estate to a charitable institution. Certain graduates (through, perhaps, their attorneys) will advise a beneficiary that a specific amount or percent of their total assets will be transferred to the institution at death.

Revocable living trusts allow donors to change their minds and alter their gift or have it returned to them. While an irrevocable arrangement is desirable, this is not as likely to occur, since donors enjoy the flexibility to make changes should their life situation be altered.

Income-producing donations such as charitable remainder trusts (unitrusts and annuity trusts) and gift annuities provide income (in the form of interest) for the donor and/or designee until they are terminated, whereupon the institution receives the principal.

Real estate remainder gifts allow donors to retain all lifetime rights to their primary residence, vacation home, or farm and to receive a charitable tax deduction. The designated charity then assumes ownership of the property after the donor's death.

Life insurance policies no longer needed for their original purpose can be given to an institution. For non-paid-up policies where premiums remain, the donor can make payment and use this as a tax deduction. If the recipient of the policy pays the premium, this amount is subtracted from the cash surrender value of the policy.

Qualified retirement plans (401K and IRA) are a way of providing a testamentary gift. By listing a charitable institution as the beneficiary on the designation form, the donor's estate will benefit from a reduction in estate and income taxes. These funds are not, however, beneficial as lifetime gifts.

To obtain planned gifts, it is typically necessary for the fund-raiser to apply a process consisting of four carefully planned steps. Each step is crucial to obtaining the desired gift. *Research* must be done to identify those graduates and friends who appear to have the capacity of making donations in excess of $25,000. The creation of a pool of major-gift prospects will be facilitated by using a MIS in conjunction with econometrics tools such as a Prospect Information Network (PIN). Following exhaustive research and a "capacity to contribute" rating conducted by the development staff, faculty, and visiting committee, the list is reduced to a palatable number of major-gift prospects. During this phase, the researchers should be concerned only with capacity to give, not propensity.

Cultivation is a process of getting to know the donor (and vice versa), building mutual trust, and determining the prospect's interests in the program. During this period (which may range from months to years), the prospect should be showered with attention and gifts. This might include flowers for a special event, tickets for the homecoming football game, an invitation to speak at a student convocation on campus, dinner at a five-star restaurant, or all of the above. During the time spent with the prospect, it is absolutely imperative to talk little and listen attentively. When you do talk, you should always try to extol the virtues of the institution and its programs. Careful listening will often help you determine with greater accuracy a prospect's capacity to give and propensity to donate to a specific program.

Solicitation of gifts must be done by the right person at the right time for the right amount and for the right purpose. The person making the request should have a close relationship with the prospect. For gift requests in excess of $100,000, I have always asked the university president to accompany me at the actual request meeting. Timing is important; asking too soon can be detrimental. The amount of the request should be realistic (based on research), yet still make the prospect flinch; under-asking can be worse than over-asking. The purpose of the request should be derived from a personalized planned-giving proposal that acknowledges the prospect's interest in a specific program or activity.

Stewardship requires the institution to use the gift in a responsible manner, whether the donation is restricted to a cause or discretionary. Celebrate each gift with appropriate "pomp and circumstance." For example, if a $100,000 donation merits a classroom being named after the donor, you should plan an appropriate dedication ceremony. Other examples include inviting the donor to the campus to observe the program of interest, to meet the scholarship recipient, or to attend a "celebration" lecture by the faculty member occupying the endowed chair. Once the gift has been used, a detailed written report of its use must be presented to the donor. Remember, donors continue to donate to causes in which their gifts have made a difference.

Lessons learned. In order to increase the likelihood of obtaining a planned gift from a prospective donor, the following lessons should be heeded:

1. Every graduate is a prospective donor; do not be misled by a person's position, car, house, or clothes. Major planned gifts do, on occasion, come from alumni living in middle-class neighborhoods.

2. Cultivation is costly in terms of money and time. Yet rarely does a major planned gift come as a result of a single contact.

3. If you seek average gifts, you are likely to receive average gifts. If the prospective donor's perceived capacity indicates that a major gift is possible, go for the gold. Do not immediately settle for a lesser gift without having made a case for a larger amount.

4. Major gifts are given to programs with a plan for future growth and development. They are seen as an investment of sorts; they are not given because a program is in financial jeopardy.

5. The right person must do the cultivation and solicitation. This person is the one who establishes a relationship of trust and respect with the prospective donor.

A planned gift is generally the result of the fund-raiser having appropriately cultivated and solicited the prospective donor. There are many creative ways in which these gifts can be beneficial to both the donor and the institution. The key to finding the most suitable gift is to seek the counsel of qualified financial planners.

Capital Campaign

A capital campaign is a cost-effective means for an institution to raise a large sum of money (often in the range of seven to nine figures) over an extended period of time (usually three to five years) for specified areas of support. These might include building construction and renovation, endowed chairs, library enhancements, faculty research funds, instructional development, and special projects. At the program level, the revenue goal is considerably smaller (usually $2-6 million) and the support areas are highly specific (e.g., develop a wellness center; equip the computer laboratory; endow undergraduate scholarships, graduate teaching/research assistantships, and professorships). For a capital campaign to be successful, it is imperative that the institution adhere to various development stages.

A typical capital campaign has seven stages. Each has a specific purpose and is critical to the success of the campaign. The *preliminary stage* begins with the institution determining that there is a need for a capital campaign. This results from a summation of the specific capital needs (or wish list) of the academic program areas. Immediately thereafter, a master plan is developed to determine the financial scope of the campaign and the institution's ability to successfully conduct it. The latter determination is often made by outside, unbiased, professional fundraising consultants. At the same time, contact is made with potential leadership gift contributors to seek their counsel on the feasibility of the campaign and to determine their willingness to be an integral part of the campaign.

A critical aspect of this initial stage is the determination of propriety for potential major gifts. It is critical that there be a "clearinghouse" (usually the officers of the foundation) to review and then assign propriety to a single institutional entity for those donors with multiple institutional interests and/or affiliations. No one in the upper echelons of administration wants to be surprised to find that an individual college, school, or department is soliciting money (usually a smaller amount) from a potential major contributor to the institution.

Testing the water requires the following: formation of an advisory committee; joint determination between the advisory committee and the institution of a realistic goal for the campaign; a firm commitment of money from leadership gift contributors (including both private and corporate agencies); preparation of a case statement articulating the institution's mission and objective for the campaign (including priority needs for funding); procurement of staff; and assemblage of volunteers who have made a firm financial commitment to the campaign.

Internal preparation includes: the development of campaign materials; the selection of major-gift prospects and the rating of their giving capacity; the assignment of prospects to a specific academic area or to a specific campaign interest area (e.g., the library, athletics); and the development of a long-range master plan detailing timelines for each campaign activity.

The in-house campaign among the institution's family (including faculty, staff, and advisory committee members) is critical to a successful campaign. Their early support aids in promoting the campaign when it is extended beyond the bounds of the institution.

Advanced gifts during this "quiet" phase are the result of the solicitation of major leadership gifts from graduates, friends, and corporations. These gifts must be finalized before the public announcement of the campaign is made and should amount to 50-to-60 percent of the campaign total.

Public solicitation is a concentrated effort on the part of the campaign staff and volunteers to conduct a campaign with broad-based appeal. This is necessary to give every potential contributor the opportunity to participate. Obviously, it is not possible to meet face to face with each potential contributor. Therefore, this phase of the campaign includes direct-mail solicitation in which a case statement and a response form are mailed to those who have not been contacted personally. It is likely that only a small number of major planned gifts will result from this stage. Potential major-gift contributors who had not been identified previously do, however, come out of the woodwork on occasion and request a personal visitation.

Wrap-up includes following up on multi-year pledges and attending to the details associated with a designated gift. Most important, it is a time to celebrate a successful campaign and to recognize both the volunteers and the contributors.

A capital campaign requires considerable institutional preparation (e.g., planning the campaign and identifying and cultivating prospective donors) and broad-based participation of volunteers in the solicitation phase. Such a campaign occurs only occasionally in the history of an institution. Thus, it is imperative that there be appropriate advanced planning. If this has occurred, it is likely that the campaign goal will not only be achieved, but surpassed.

Lessons learned. For capital campaigns to be successful, fund-raisers are encouraged to adhere to the following guidelines:

1. The case statement for the campaign must be embraced by the campaign staff (including volunteers) and the prospective contributors.
2. A "top down" donor pyramid will identify levels of giving and the number of gifts at each level that must be secured. It is imperative to understand that approximately 80 percent of the campaign goal will come from 20 percent of the contributors. These individuals are identified at the upper level of the pyramid. Therefore, for a $10 million campaign goal to be achieved, there will need to be at least one gift of $1,000,000, two of $750,000, four at $500,000, and so on. People without capital-campaign experience are likely to suggest finding 1,000 people who will give $10,000. This is virtually impossible.

Thus, successful campaigns focus most of their time, effort, and finances on obtaining gifts from the upper echelons of the donor population (i.e., those with the capacity to make a major gift).

3. Volunteer leaders who are committed to the campaign and who have made a financial contribution to it are imperative. Others will follow their lead.

4. Timing for the campaign must be right. A prematurely initiated campaign will likely result in failure.

5. Institutions must direct campaign gifts to their intended beneficiaries and be good stewards of such gifts. This will likely result in future contributions.

6. Donor recognition is imperative and must reflect the institution's appreciation. Examples include naming a building, classroom, professorship, or scholarship after the donor; bestowing an appropriate plaque; or simply offering a personal thank you.

A capital campaign is a means of ensuring financial security and growth for institutions and promising programs that would not be possible if they relied solely on their appropriated budget. Such a campaign makes it possible for them to achieve prominence.

Summary

One of the biggest challenges facing higher-education institutions is obtaining sufficient funding to adequately support academic programs. Most administrators have become reconciled to the fact that their appropriated budgets are inadequate, and that extramural funding must be sought from alumni, friends, corporations, and foundations. Unfortunately, many administrators and faculty are still reluctant to seek such funding. Administrators associated with the College and University Administrators Council of the American Alliance for Health, Physical Education, Recreation, and Dance are an exception. They are endeavoring to provide programs, workshops, and publications on fundraising for the benefit of those among their ranks who are committed to the enhancement of their programs through the generation of extramural resources.

An anonymous writer once wrote, "Money is not given, it is to be raised. Money is not offered, it has to be asked for. Money does not come in, it must be gone after" (Lord, 1988, p. 113). It is the intent of this writing to further acquaint HPERD personnel with the art and science of "going after" extra funds by reaching out to alumni. Many of the challenges facing fund-raisers have been identified and described in detail in James F. Greenfield's (1999) *Fund Raising: Evaluating and Managing the Fund-Development Process.* Notable among these challenges are accountability, cost-effectiveness, ethics, outcomes measurement, volunteers, and women in philanthropy.

The single most pressing challenge for HPERD personnel is to initiate efforts to "go after" extramural monies. It is possible to have successful annual funds drives, to obtain major planned gifts, and to conduct a capital campaign. What do you see in the following letters: *OPPORTUNITIES-ARENOWHERE?* Those who are pessimistic about fundraising success are certain that "opportunities are nowhere"; those who have successful experience in raising extramural funds are certain that "opportunities are now here." Frankly, the opportunities are everywhere. The requests, however, must be made. The place to begin is with the alumni.

About the Author

J. William Douglas, professor and dean emeritus in the School of Physical Education at West Virginia University, has been engaged in fundraising and alumni relations for 21 years. In May 2001, he will retire after 41 years in higher education as a teacher, coach, administrator, and fund-raiser.

References

Burdinski, R. A. (2000). Proceed according to plan. *Currents, 26*(5), 19-22.

Greenfield, J. M. (1999). *Fund raising: Evaluating and managing the fund-development process* (2nd ed.). New York: John Wiley & Sons.

Lord, J. G. (1998). *The raising of money: Thirty-five essentials every trustee should know.* Cleveland, OH: Third Sector Press.

Sharpe, R. F. (1999). *Planned giving simplified: The gift, the giver, and the gift planner.* New York: John Wiley & Sons.

18 Developing and Managing a Balanced Budget

Trent Gabert, *Associate Dean, College of Liberal Studies, University of Oklahoma*

The buck stops here.

— President Harry S. Truman

The development and management of university financial concerns must begin with the mission, vision, goals, and objectives of the institution and of the units within it (colleges, departments, programs). Philosophically speaking, a democratic approach to developing and managing finances will more likely lead to commitment and optimal effectiveness from each person within the unit, at least in the short run. The early-to-mid-20th-century autocratic processes of leadership and management have evolved into a more desirable format involving increased representation of all stakeholders through the use of budgetary teams, public review, open records, and attention to employee and customer demands for fairness, equity, and accountability.

Budget Basics   A budget is a detailed schedule of financial activities (e.g., marketing expenditures for the recruitment of high-quality students; resources and expenditures on research grants; the day-to-day operation of a unit). A budget is a part of a larger financial plan that includes strategic financial objectives, assumptions, strategies, contingency plans, and a period-by-period program for financing an entire operation (Emmery & Finnerty, 1997). Total financial planning seldom occurs effectively in small units (e.g., a health, physical education, recreation, or dance [HPERD] department) because a very high percentage of their monies are tied directly to salaries and wages and very little flexibility is available for shifting large portions to a different category. Within a larger unit (e.g., a school or college), however, financial planning is needed so that effective differential financing can take place. For example, when such a unit is making significant downward budget adjustments, a decision must be made about how the reduction will be implemented (e.g., across-the-board proportional

173

cuts, vertical cuts, variable cuts). The same may be true when new monies need to be distributed.

Budgets have two main purposes (Bryan, 1998). First, they help measure the financial commitment needed to support the activities that are necessary for reaching stated goals. For example, how much money must be allocated to the health-promotion degree program in order to improve its internship opportunities? Second, budgets serve as an important internal control that can alert management to changes in operating effectiveness. Thus, budgets are the standards often used to measure progress in achieving unit goals and objectives. For example, if no change occurs in the funded internship program, then the budget allows one to decide if the allocation has been a waste of resources.

Barber (1996) listed several practical advantages of budgeting:

1. It substitutes a plan for chance in fiscal operations by foreseeing expenditure needs; it also organizes staff, along with the work that needs to be accomplished.
2. It requires review of the entire operation (all divisions and subdivisions) in terms of available funds and revenue needs; it prevents over-budgeting (padding).
3. It promotes standardization and simplification of operation by establishing priorities and objectives, and it eliminates inefficient operations.
4. It provides guidelines for staff to follow and acts as an instrument for fiscal control.
5. It gives the governing body factual data for evaluating the efficiency of the operation.
6. It helps the taxpaying public and other contributors see where revenues are coming from and how they are being used.

To connect the means and ends, budgets must be developed by those responsible for the attainment of the stated goals and objectives and fully communicated to those responsible for their approval. Therefore, budgets should be developed by faculty teams and approved by the governing board, director, or dean. Budgetary teams provide an increased level of input for effective processing, a stronger identification of internal needs and external resources, and a check-and-balance system. Under strong autocratic or laissez-faire management, the budget process is more susceptible to human error. The functional composition of a budgetary team should include expertise, representation, experience, action, and forward thinking. Faculty budgetary teams give representation to smaller sub-units, in effect providing communication channels within the system. Budgetary teams also allow for more complete commitment from more individuals to the entire budgetary process. In addition to commitment, budget activities require both short and long-term action planning. Therefore, small teams may better meet short-term needs, while larger teams (never more then five to nine members) may better meet long-term needs.

Budgets, developed as a part of the strategic-planning process, are really no more than operational plans expressed in financial terms. However, in addition to this strict business formula, budgets are about values: "We express the connection between money and values every time we tell someone that 'talk is cheap' and it is time to 'put your money where your mouth is'" (Cozzetto, Kweit, & Kweit, 1995). In this sense, budgeting is much more then mere financial statements. In fact, Guthrie, Garms, and Pierce (1988) asserted that school budgeting is not the same as business budgeting. For schools, budgeting: (1) is more usefully viewed as a component of management's planning and evaluation activities; (2) should represent a plan for directing an organization's total discretionary resources (e.g., time, personnel, physical resources), not simply money; and (3) must be understood as a political activity, not simply a technocratic undertaking. In fact, Cozzetto et al. indicated that only the accurate record-keeping is a technical activity. Before any record-keeping, budget decisions in educational organizations involve significant bargaining and value orientations about equality, efficiency, good faith, and organizational outcomes. It is through budgeting that an organization aligns its resources with its purposes (Guthrie et al.). The budget process is also the concrete link between the planning stage of an organization's management activities, the forward-looking stage, and the evaluation stage, which focuses systematically on past performances.

While a simple budget may consist of an estimate of receipts and payments for a period of time, it is also important as a predictive tool. A budget team can anticipate the flow of revenues and expenditures. In this sense, a budget is a guide to the financial expectations of a unit and an expression of management's plans (Garrison, 1982).

For budgeting to be most effective, three critical conditions should exist: annularity, comprehensiveness, and balance (Wildavsky, 1984). Annularity refers to a budget as an organization's resource allocation plan that is intended to cover a fixed period, generally a year. The budget year is generally known as a fiscal year; for many American schools, the fiscal year begins on July 1 and concludes at the end of the following June, in the next calendar year. However, some institutions begin the fiscal year as the start of the school year, while others use a two-year period. The dates that are used are most often determined by state budgetary policy. To optimize efficiency in the budget process, constancy in start and end dates is important; otherwise, public confidence, record-keeping, and fiscal analyses are often jeopardized.

Fundamental Components of Budgeting

Comprehensiveness means that an organization's budget should encompass all fiscal activity, on both the resource and expenditure sides. The budget process must encompass all revenues received by an organization and all its expenditures, regardless of their source or purpose. If a budget is not comprehensive, organizational resources may be accrued or used for purposes outside its management team's control. This may or may not be illegal, but it is very often inefficient, and disruptive to other members of the organization.

Balance is also crucial; what is received by way of resources must not exceed what is spent. This is not to assert that all organizations must always live within their immediately available resources. Certainly resources can be borrowed and paid back later. Borrowing monies to construct a long-lasting facility makes good sense. The point is that a budget assumes explicit organizational acknowledgement of resources and obligations, and the two must match. If they are out of balance, an organization is out of control.

Mission, Vision, Goals, and Objectives

To produce meaningful budgets, an organization must periodically review its mission statement. A subset of the budget team needs to be held responsible for this annual review. If a unit does not understand and communicate its mission, vision, goals, and objectives, then it will not know where it is headed, and even the best budget will not help it get there!

The preparation of a budget begins with the establishment or review of the mission, vision, goals, and objectives. A quick review of these critical concepts is important. The mission is what an organization represents and attempts to achieve. In our discipline, we attempt to provide quality educational programs, conduct research, and serve various constituencies in the areas of dance, exercise, health, recreation, and sport. Few management sources, especially in our literature, describe vision. However, it is a very important part of the recent literature on leadership. A vision is a new direction or emphasis for an organization (Nanus, 1992). It is a plan that is set forth for a two-to-five-year period. Examples of a vision include the elimination of an undergraduate program, the development of a new graduate emphasis within any one of the areas listed under the mission statement, a concerted effort to raise employee salaries, and improved service in helping students attain internships and jobs. A vision is a well-thought-out plan, but it is through the goals and objectives that the vision is realized.

Goals are the specific elements within the mission and vision that hold all action to a particular standard of quality and achievement. Goals serve as elements for evaluation and guide both the organization and its employees in reaching the mission and vision. For example, related HPERD goals may be the development of a PhD specialization in sport law, within a three-year timeframe, for the sport-management program (Nanus, 1992). Several goals make up the vision. Objectives are the steps that are necessary to achieve the goals. In the above example of developing a new PhD program, objectives may include a needs assessment, program development, and recruiting of qualified faculty.

Developing a Budget

Budget development embodies a concern for what will or should be. Most budget planning may be discussed in terms of the four phases that make up the budget cycle: (1) preparation, (2) presentation, (3) adoption, execution, and post-execution, and (4) audit (Guthrie et al., 1988).

Budgets contain factors such as fixed costs, state appropriations, variable income-generating programs, "soft" monies, salaries/wages (e.g., for faculty, staff, students), promotions, fringe benefits, supplies, travel, equipment, communication, marketing, public relations, maintenance, technology development/usage, surplus, and, sometimes, depreciation. While the format of most budget processes is highly influenced by organizational, state, and federal regulations, a good budget leader will try to optimize flexibility whenever possible, provided that it is for the good of the unit, personnel within the unit, and students. Flexibility allows the budget-management teams to shift resources based on growth and helps them enact visionary planning, new goals and objectives, and—though undesirable or unforeseen—reductions in specific areas (if revenues decrease precipitously over time). Clearly, budgetary effectiveness involves much more than bookkeeping, although that is a critical element in the process.

Budget development is the actual preparation of financial data, which requires a review of past budget items and of the unit's vision, goals, and objectives. This review should result in a document that will eventually be presented to the leadership and accepted for a period of time. This document will include information in all areas of income, expenses, surplus, etc., and may show comparisons with the budget from the previous fiscal year. The presentation of a draft is a political process. Therefore, the draft should be legitimate, supported by major or minor entities within the organization, and presented enthusiastically to management. The draft should be clear and precise, and include supporting documentation, statistics, charts, need statements, and so forth. Supporting documentation is especially important during periods of change in the unit's direction, given the resultant reallocation of resources. Key personnel should review the draft several times and then present it to all members of the unit in an open forum. This of course depends on the content of the budget, as salary data is seldom discussed in an open forum. Following discussion, the document should be ready for approval, followed by interpretation and execution.

The development of a budget requires a budget calendar. Chronological events and issues (e.g., university-required equipment proposals and salary recommendations; beginning of a fiscal year; time lag in gaining equipment approval) must be understood in terms of this calendar. The length of time that a budget covers depends on institutional, state, and federal guidelines. Again, most budgets operate on an annual basis, while others may be set up for a two-year period. The overall objective of the entire budget process is to end up with a well-balanced program for the unit; this program will in turn serve as the core justification for requested resources (Rabin, Hildreth, & Miller, 1996).

We know that emergencies (and, occasionally, windfalls) are bound to occur. Leaders who plan ahead can activate special budget requests more easily when necessary. For example, an institution may suddenly ask a unit what it needs in the way of technology upgrades. If the unit must take the time to assess its needs before answering, then it may be too late in firing off its proposal to central administration. A good budget calendar always plans for annually recurring events, but it should also have a long and creative needs-assessment section that allows the unit to respond quickly to unexpected requests. It is also advisable for the budget team to annually prioritize this needs list so that leadership can react immediately: never miss out when unexpected resources appear!

In addition to budget events, a calendar should include a connecting column that lists who should participate in the discussion for each event. Some units have separate groups that handle salary increases (usually a committee representing experienced faculty), research equipment (a committee made up of key researchers who clearly understand equipment needs), and so forth. The listing of discussion participants can help an administrator gain immediate information from appropriate faculty and staff and then quickly respond to central administration.

Significant effort and time must also be expended to garner financial resources. This will occur most effectively if the process is planned, the needs of individuals and programs are considered, and a semi-formal team environment is fostered. The process will also be enhanced if goals are clearly stated. Seldom are monies given, distributed, or reallocated without important, clearly expressed, and often politically motivated goal statements. Budgetary teams should spend sufficient time developing and understanding goals before even attempting to develop a budget.

Important steps in this process include: generating income from grant activities, private donations, and fundraising events; securing a fair share of the unit's budget; and demonstrating careful cost-containment measures. Budgetary effectiveness will be lessened without careful consideration of each of these elements in relation to each other. In this sense, the budget becomes a system, or a reactionary process, in that what happens in one part of the budget will necessarily have an effect on another part of the process.

Often, the cost of generating revenue cannot be measured solely in terms of dollars; the time taken away from teaching, research, and service when a unit ventures into new capital areas must also be considered as a cost. It is also important to consider that while any new venture will have its costs, they may well be worthwhile in the long run. One must take calculated risks to move forward. In addition, the psychological benefit derived from the challenge of garnering resources can greatly enhance team building and commitment among diverse portions of a unit.

After the budget is adopted, it is the responsibility of senior management (chair, director, dean) to administer it. Periodic meetings by the budget team will be important in determining if allocations are allowing goals to be met, if the monies assigned to objectives are being used appropriately, and if any adjustments to the budget need to be made. While certain budget limits are carved in stone, the budget should be flexible enough to allow for accommodations. Substantial shifts in goals and objectives may require review and revision of the budget. However, the prime directive of any budget, regardless of potential alterations, is to achieve the mission, vision, goals, and objectives established at the outset of the process. Thus, the review procedure involves evaluating whether or not all budget assumptions were achieved and the mission fulfilled. If a unit is large, a business manager may be assigned the task of tracking the budget. This person will be very important in helping the budget team by: providing records and analyses; maintaining and monitoring paperwork on personnel, purchases, and bid requests; participating in budget development for grants; and so forth.

Finally, an audit must be performed in order to ensure that monies are accounted for according to the preparation, adoption, and execution stages of the budget process. During the audit portion of any budgeting situation, it is critical that the unit adhere to fiscal limitations. Overspending or under-spending without documentation, justification, and approval is unacceptable. Therefore, the audit is the evaluation process that determines the level of success of the present year's budget and serves as the basis for the next year's budget.

Accounting

Accounting is a disclosure review involving several components (Barber, 1996). First is managerial or internal accounting that is based on projections from the adopted budget. Managerial accounting verifies that monies are collected and dispensed according to the adopted plan. This is a primary influence on management's decision-making efforts. Tracking accrued actual expenditures and encumbrances—resources that have already been obligated though not spent—are important parts of managerial accounting. This procedure must be kept current and reviewed by management on a monthly basis. It is suggested that the budget team meet and review the internal account reports and then assist with changes or revisions if necessary.

External account reports primarily involve an income statement, a balance sheet, and a cash-flow statement. These reports are subject to independent internal or external auditing, sometimes annually, but more often every few years. It is better to be over-informed and safe than under-informed and irresponsible. External accounts must conform to the generally accepted accounting procedures of the larger organization (e.g., university, state). It is important that these accounts be objective and unbiased because the confidence of the campus and public is at stake. Lack of confidence either internally or externally will almost always increase the difficulty of garnering resources in the future.

Financial record-keeping helps a unit use past information as the basis for future financial analyses (e.g., cost-effectiveness analysis or appraisals of equity). Specific, categorized information is extremely valuable in analyzing budget issues. For example, a single, general category for "equipment" will not be of much use when one is looking to analyze a unit's golf expenditures over a five-year period. Categorical analyses are especially important for self-supporting activities within a unit. For example, we ran a highly successful adult-fitness program in our department for many years. The many goals of the program included fitness education, fitness assessment, and actual classes. We found that we lost money in several categories, while the actual classes made so much money that they provided a surplus, supporting research assistants and equipment for many areas of the department. Because of our analyses, the budget team soon realized that unless the insolvent activities were used for research purposes, they were not financially viable parts of the operation.

This last example demonstrates another important part of accounting: cost-benefit analysis. Cost-benefit analyses allow budget teams to decide whether the value obtained from certain cost-loss activities is important enough that they should be retained when the overall operation is cost-effective. Some items are psychologically important, as was the case in our adult-fitness-education programs. The budget team decided that even though no monies were generated from these specific activities, they were extremely valuable in recruiting faculty, staff, and community members for our paid classes and research projects, and they were a great public outreach for key personnel across campus. Cost-benefit analysis can also help justify important courses with low enrollment. If you can show that higher enrollment in some popular courses offsets the losses in other low-enrollment (but very important) courses, then you have a much stronger basis for argument than just stating, "Well, these courses are important and we need to offer them." Another form of cost-benefit analysis involves investigating the income and costs associated with different class and lab arrangements. Which is the better arrangement: having a key faculty member teaching two classes of 30 students, each with its own lab section, or having a large lecture for 60 students taught by the professor, with three lab sections taught by a graduate assistant? One must determine not only the economics of such arrangements, but also the comparative quality of instruction, space, graduate-assistant support, faculty mentoring of graduate assistants, and so forth. There may be little difference in cost between the two arrangements, but the connections established between key faculty members and graduate assistants and the development of graduate assistants as entry-level lecturers may be invaluable in the long run.

Administration of a Budget

Several types of budgeting are quite common in HPERD units. The easiest to understand and most common type is "object-classification budgeting." This form of budgeting defines the areas of expense and income in a uniform grouping of categories. One common format—which may be part of the software package used at your institution or could be created by hand—might include the following categories (Barber, 1996):

Expenses	Income
1000 Services: Personnel	**1000 State Monies**
1100 Salaries, regular	1100 Salaries, regular
1110 Administration	1110 Administration
1120 Faculty	1120 Faculty
1130 Staff	1130 Staff
1200 Salaries, temporary	1200 Salaries, temporary
1210 Graduate assistants	1210 Graduate assistants
1300 Wages, regular	1300 Wages, regular
1400 Wages, temporary	1400 Wages, temporary
1410 Teaching	1410 Teaching
1420 Student	1420 Student
1430 Staff	**2000 Contractual**
1500 Other compensations	2010 Telephone
1510 Retirement	2020 Postage
1511 TIAA	2030 Equipment
1520 Health insurance	**3000 Travel**
1530 Dental insurance	**4000 Non-State Monies**
1540 Life insurance	4010 Special course fees
2000 Services: Contractual	4020 Donations
2100 Communication	4021 Telethon
2110 Telephone	4022 Annual alumni
2120 Computer	4030 Grant monies

The above is only a partial list; it can be expanded or altered to meet the needs of any unit. At the same time, it is uniform, easy to set up and manage, and very clear and straightforward. Furthermore, this type of budget is common among many different organizations, thus easing the learning curve for current and future personnel.

A second oft-used form of budgeting is "line-item budgeting." This is very similar to the object-classification format, but instead of listing a category by number, lines are identified by name. Early versions of this format listed every item, but general names are used today (e.g., "recreational sport supplies," "office supplies").

A third form of budgeting is the "program budget," which separates an organization into unique units. A program budget could easily be adopted by a HPERD department. Generally, there are three components to such a budget: sub-unit goals, program goals, and unique features of the sub-unit and its programs. Identification of these components is then followed by a line-item or object-classification budget. Each sub-portion of an academic department would develop a separate budget, with a narrative description of its program goals and objectives. Priorities should be established in this narrative to show special emphases that can then be reviewed by the budget team and compared across all sub-units. The descriptive narrative provides much more value orientation than numbers and lines.

Performance budgeting is very similar to the program-budget process. However, it also includes a description of what services are provided by the institution, not just how much money is being spent. Categories within the performance model are defined by the amount of time that is required to perform the activity. Then, a cost can be attributed to each activity. The manager has a great deal of financial control and can be precise when using this type of budget.

A planning programming budget system (PPBS) is another useful form of budgeting. The focus of this format is on the end product of the service provided rather than on the actual cost. One of the purposes of a PPBS is to provide a rationale for each of the competing budget items within a department or college. This technique is very helpful when resources are limited.

Zero-based budgeting is based on the premise that an organization begins each year with no money. In this form, a budget is prepared by justifying each expenditure as if it were a new expense. The purpose of this type of budget is to control overbudgeting and waste. The leadership has to scrutinize the reasonableness of every budget request in relation to the entire organization. This form is helpful in breaking from traditional methods in which allocations are made with little regard to new needs and changes over time.

There are many other (less frequently used) forms of budgeting. Increment-decrement budgeting increases or decreases the percentage for each item over time. This is a good form to use when developing long-term budgets. Capital budget planning describes capital expenses that include long-range budget items. A capital budget often covers a longer period (perhaps up to 10 years) and includes major purchases that are not usually found in annual operating budgets. Capital budgets also require a narrative and a clear justification for use and need. The enterprise-fund system of budgeting works on the premise that every individual program within an organization is its own separate enterprise. The revenue generated by a given program is thus used to finance that program's operation. The underlying assumption in enterprise systems is that enterprises will generate a profit; in a flexible system, this profit may be classified as "draw-on-next-year" funds or be used to fund other enterprises within the organization. Not all portions of an organization will be self-sufficient; thus, the profits from one enterprise can be used to shore up another area. Each of the above forms of budgeting has been modified from Barber (1996); when developing any one of these forms, the reader should review this source.

Budgeting, Decision-Making, and Power

Individuals empowered to make decisions regarding resource allocation can determine an organization's direction. Frankly, budget control equals organizational control or, more simply, power (Guthrie et al., 1988). The budget process can be used to concentrate power in the hands of a relatively small number of individuals or to distribute it to an expanded number of areas. To understand this process, we must understand the incremental nature of budgeting; the tendency of most any budget team is to make resource-allocation changes only at the margins. The vast majority of expenditures are the same year after year, budget cycle after budget cycle; the base changes very little. The main reason for this is the political influence of individuals and groups that benefit from the status quo. Faculty and the programs they serve want as many of the new resources as possible, should there be any available. Faculty raises, new faculty to teach added sections, and new equipment to serve existing faculty needs are just a few of the typical demands. Consequently, the budget team is under tremendous political pressure to resist significant change, and therefore to support the mainstream of the organization. Faculty representing existing programs desire a fair portion of new monies and are very protective against any cuts that may occur in favor of new programs. In such an environment, the best that one can hope for is an addition to the base.

Several techniques can be used to help a unit move away from incremental budgeting. PPBS, management by objectives (MBO), and zero-based budgeting are particularly helpful. Each of these processes calls for resources to be aligned with organizational purposes, programs, or objectives, instead of with actual objects to be purchased, personnel, and materials. If a purpose is agreed on by the decision-makers, then expenditures necessary to accomplish this purpose are permitted. If a purpose or program is no longer thought to be fundamentally important, then its expenditure base is reduced or eliminated. Thus, an old purpose or program may be replaced by a new one. Although PPBS and MOB initially appear to be more centralized, or "top-down," than team budgeting, there really is no reason why these processes cannot be decentralized and connected to a zero-based process from the bottom up. In this scenario, budgets are initially determined at the level where objectives are carried out, and then the process flows up to the budget team. When budget needs reach the top, reviews and decisions must be made to match these needs with the overall organizational budget. This is another means for the budget team to review goals and objectives and offer support for those units best supporting the vision and mission of the organization. In a practical sense, the personnel responsible for the objectives must periodically submit two budget requests: one below their need levels and one above them. This helps the budget team make decisions about elimination or reduction if necessary. As much as one may like zero-based budgeting, it must be remembered that only a fraction of a typical budget is actually flexible enough for change to take place. Most monies are connected to fixed factors such as salaries and fringe benefits. This is why fundraising, donations, "soft" monies, and so forth are so beneficial to units—they allow change to occur!

Summary

Whatever budgeting system is employed, there must be a strong connection between the resultant budget and the mission, vision, goals, and objectives of the unit. Thus a team process in budgeting is particularly valuable, as it ensures representation for all members of the unit while at the same time maintaining accountability in the budget process.

About the Author

Trent Gabert is the associate dean of the College of Liberal Studies at the University of Oklahoma. Before becoming associate dean, he served as chair of the Department of Health and Sport Sciences for 14 years. He is currently completing his 31st year at the University of Oklahoma.

References

Barber, E. (1996). Accounting and budgeting. In B.L. Parkhouse (Ed.), *The management of sport: Its foundation and application* (pp. 343-362). St. Louis, MO: Mosby.

Bryan, R. M. (1998). The basics of budgeting: Your role in developing a meaningful budget. *Association Management, 50*(1), 65-67.

Cozzetto, D. A., Kweit, M. G., & Kweit, R. W. (1995). *Public budgeting: Politics, institutions, and processes*. White Plains, NY: Longman.

Emmery, D. R., & Finnerty, J. D. (1997). *Corporate financial management*. Upper Saddle River, NJ: Prentice-Hall.

Garrison, R. (1982). *Managerial accounting*. Plano, TX: Business Publications.

Guthrie, J. W., Garms, W. I., & Pierce, L. C. (1988). *School finance and education policy: Enhancing educational efficiency, equality, and choice*. Englewood Cliffs, NJ: Prentice-Hall.

Nanus, B. (1992). *Visionary leadership: Creating a compelling sense of direction for your organization*. San Francisco: Jossey-Bass.

Parkhouse, B. L. (1996). *The management of sport: Its foundation and application*. St. Louis: Mosby.

Rabin, J., Hildreth, W. B., & Miller, G. J. (1996). *Budgeting: Formulation and execution*. Athens, GA: The Carl Vinson Institute of Government.

Wildavsky, A. (1984). *The politics of the budgetary process*. Boston: Little Brown.

SECTION IV

Outside Agencies

19 Establishing Partnerships within the Community

Garth Tymeson, *Professor and Interim Dean, College of Health, Physical Education, Recreation, and Teacher Education, University of Wisconsin–La Crosse*

All the money in the world cannot solve problems unless we work together. And, if we work together, there is no problem in the world that can stop us as we seek to develop people to their highest potential.

⊶ Ewing Marion Kauffman

More and more, colleges and universities are expected to expand their mission and direct their impact beyond the walls of campus classrooms. As this occurs, partnerships with community constituencies of all types become necessary. These collaborative relationships should be mutually beneficial and provide professional growth opportunities for all involved. Administrators must possess the knowledge and skills to establish successful partnerships with community agencies in order to accomplish goals such as cutting costs, developing student and faculty learning opportunities, increasing revenues, and enhancing public relations for their units.

Expanded missions and services developed through partnerships result in additional and challenging roles and responsibilities for administrators (Stoel, Togneri, & Brown, 1992). These new roles must be recognized, accepted, and developed if health, physical education, recreation, and dance (HPERD) units are to survive and flourish in a more complex, competitive, and collaborative higher-education arena. Expansion beyond the familiarity of campuses and traditional roles leads to many positive outcomes for colleges and universities and their collaborators. Administrators need to take advantage of these opportunities to highlight the many contributions that HPERD units make to the "big picture" on campus and in surrounding communities. A unit that does not establish partnerships with community agencies risks being viewed as "old school" and unable to meet the demands and realities of the present.

Administrators often serve as initial facilitators and ongoing managers for the development of partnerships with the external community; if not, they can at least serve as resources for those attempting to form such partnerships. Historically, HPERD units have often been campus leaders in community involvement (O'Sullivan, Tannehill, Knop, Pope, & Henninger, 1999) and have reaped many political, financial, and other rewards as a result of serving external constituencies. Common partnerships and services implemented by HPERD units have included sports camps, recreation programs, clinical fieldwork or internship experiences for future professionals, and provision of inservice education or other professional development for community-based programs and professionals. We need to expand such collaboration and take advantage of the expertise and resources that our units possess to serve community partners. Colleges and universities are very visible community residents, and this status must be used as a means of assisting with partnership ventures.

This chapter offers an overview of community partnerships for HPERD units. The goal is to provide practical information to current and future administrators that can help them develop and implement positive community-relations activities that lead to mutually beneficial partnerships. Detailed information is presented regarding the reasons for developing partnerships, suggested community partners, how to establish and maintain partnerships, assessment guidelines, and examples of successful partnerships.

Why Establish Partnerships?

As time, effort, and resource demands increase in all aspects of higher education, it is important to understand why partnerships are worth pursuing. Unless there are demonstrated and agreed-upon benefits to be gained from these activities, it would be unwise for administrators and other personnel to spend precious time and resources on external partnerships.

Colleges and universities are integral parts of communities, however, and they must reach out to both impact and benefit from local constituencies. Specifically, partnerships can establish HPERD units as vital contributors to local communities. Units are expected to form such relationships if they are at all involved in the community. Community members should view the university as a willing supporter that aggressively works to share its resources. The bottom line is that establishing partnerships is the right thing to do.

Positive public relations can also result from successful partnerships. Administrators need to work regularly with their institution's community-relations staff to gain publicity for partnership efforts. There are many benefits to informing internal and external constituents about collaborative efforts. Such publicity often leads to more opportunities, as other agencies discover activities and goals that they have in common with your unit. Other individuals and groups will want to be part of the successful relations created by your community partnerships.

Furthermore, higher-education governing boards, central administrators, the public, and others expect academic units to expand their missions and services. HPERD units and their administrators need to be part of this expansion into the community. Don't let your unit be viewed as inflexible or unable to adjust its scope. These expanded roles and expectations are all part of the development of community collaboration.

Financial benefits can also result from partnerships. This could include direct payment for services, cost-sharing to decrease expenditures, and real savings accrued through the use of existing equipment or facilities. You may gain direct or indirect access to funds that would not be available to you if not for the partnership. For example, a public school district or county human-service agency in partnership with your unit may be able to use state or local government funds that are not typically available to your institution. Grant proposals can be written that may allow your unit to subcontract from a grantee—who may be your partner. Many funding opportunities require collaborative grant proposals or evidence of significant partnership among those who will implement and/or benefit from the grant-funded program. Foundations commonly have funding restrictions that may limit participation for certain agencies. In partnerships, these limitations may be overcome, and many more potential funding sources could be available. An example of such a situation is funding that is available to law-enforcement agencies for youth-violence prevention. Public-health and other youth-service providers in higher education could link with local police departments or other eligible public agencies to access these funds for collaborative programs.

Partnerships can also directly benefit college students in many different ways. Undergraduate and graduate students can participate in many worthwhile experiences, such as student teaching, internships, job shadowing, and research opportunities, any of which may ultimately lead to employment. Students also benefit from faculty involvement in partnerships, as faculty obtain up-to-date information about the "real world" and pass it on to students in classroom and other settings.

Other prime beneficiaries of partnerships are faculty and staff. A faculty member's teaching, service, and scholarship performance can be enhanced through involvement in appropriately structured partnerships. Exposure to external agencies provides faculty with up-to-date information and practices in their field. Opportunities for research can also be expanded through collaborative efforts. It is very common for program-efficacy studies and other types of field-based or action-research projects to evolve from community partnerships. These projects can translate into publications and or presentations, so long as all partners are included as coauthors/presenters. In addition, many faculty members are often rejuvenated through a new assignment as part of an external partnership. This can serve as an important faculty-development technique for administrators.

Partnerships also tend to result in many benefits for external agencies (e.g., for their employees and finances). These benefits are important, since time and energy will be expended on the relationships and employees will ask, "What am I or my agency getting out of this?" Several of the same benefits derived by the college or university are obtained by the agency. Experienced university administrators often report that outside agencies expect universities to have experts who can rejuvenate or update their staff. They look to universities for leadership, best practices, and cutting-edge ideas. Perhaps the most important benefit of partnerships is the positive impact they have on the community in general. Whether the partnership results in improved prevention programs, enhanced recreation, sport, and fitness opportunities, or other types of benefits, the positive influence of collaborative projects on the community is a key justification for their implementation.

Possible Partners

Communities surrounding institutions of higher education generally contain many potential partners for collaborative efforts. Administrators and faculty who are in tune with their local communities will find it easier to locate agencies with missions similar to their own. Finding such common bonds is an effective way to serve those in the community (Wilbur & Lambert, 1995). As this occurs, the range of potential partners in a community expands, and opportunities grow for HPERD units. HPERD administrators can look to the following types of agencies for potential collaboration:

- Police departments and other law-enforcement agencies
- Human service agencies such as county health departments, youth bureaus, social services, and family resources
- Public and private schools, including preschools and Head Start programs
- Professional organizations such as national, regional, state, and local affiliates of the American Heart Association, American Cancer Society, American Public Health Association, National Collegiate Athletics Association, National Recreation and Parks Association, American College of Sports Medicine, National Athletic Trainers Association, and American Alliance for Health, Physical Education, Recreation, and Dance
- Community service organizations such as Rotary Club, Optimists, Lion's Club, Knights of Columbus, Kiwanis, and American Legion
- Municipal park and recreation departments and other youth-enrichment programs
- State departments of education or public instruction, including state high school athletics associations or other relevant governing agencies
- Public, private, corporate, and community foundations
- Local, state, regional, and federal agencies (e.g., U.S. Department of Education, Department of Health and Human Services, Department of Justice)
- Hospitals, sports-medicine facilities, and other health-related or medical facilities
- Private companies and corporations
- Local YW/YMCAs, Boys' and Girls' Clubs, 4H Clubs, and other youth agencies
- Health and recreation businesses (e.g., bowling, golf, and fitness facilities)
- Church groups.

The list goes on and on. Opportunities for partnerships will vary according to the location of an institution, but no matter where you are located, there will be many agencies waiting to pursue mutually beneficial partnerships. Your challenge is to form a collaboration that will help them meet their goals.

The need for partnerships between higher education and PK-12 education was recently highlighted in a new federal grant program sponsored the U.S. Department of Education. GEAR-UP (Gaining Early Awareness and Readiness for Undergraduate Programs) provides grants to locally designed partnerships between higher education institutions, high-poverty middle schools, and at least two other organizations (e.g., community-based organizations, businesses, religious groups, state education agencies, parent groups, non-profit agencies). HPERD units could be part of these grant efforts. Administrators need to be aware of opportunities like these to become active partners in their communities. For more information on GEAR-UP and other educational-partnership grant programs, contact the National Council for Community and Education Partnerships, One Dupont Circle NW, Suite 118, Washington, DC 20036; (202) 939-9450; www.edparnterships.org. Many other public agencies have grant programs for partnerships that serve their constituents. Private foundations will almost always request information regarding collaboration and partnerships in their grant proposals.

Hastad and Tymeson (1997) have suggested a multi-step process for developing successful partnerships with external agencies. Implementation of these steps can result in successful community relations and help HPERD administrators focus their collaboration efforts. Of course, local circumstances need to be combined with these general guidelines.

How to Establish Partnerships

Identify community needs that match your strategic vision. The initial phase of developing partnerships is to identify community needs that are important to both local constituencies and your own unit, and then to analyze whether these needs could be fully or partially met through systematic, collaborative efforts. Look for potential partners with goals that are similar to yours. Familiarity with your community, direct experience in working with local agencies, and reliance on good professional judgment and creativity will all help you conduct this needs assessment. Examples of common needs that HPERD units could address include: (1) health-related fitness programs for youths and adults, (2) youth-enrichment programs of all types, (3) programs that enhance economic growth through expansions in tourism, recreation, and/or other health-related professions, (4) exercise, recreation, health-enhancement, and sport programs for individuals with disabilities, (5) sport and recreation programs for youths, (6) staff-development programs, (7) shared use of facilities, transportation, and personnel, and (8) coordination of multiple (or redundant) health, recreation, education, enrichment, and physical activity services by a central source. You will likely identify many partially or completely unmet needs in your community. As a matter of fact, most successful partnerships will lead to numerous unanticipated community-involvement opportunities (success breeds more success). When this occurs, it is important to avoid the temptation to tackle too many initiatives. The success of most collaborative efforts depends on need and on the ability to focus sustained time, resources, energies, and talents toward meeting that need. It is better to be successful at meeting one need and building on that accomplishment than to inadequately address multiple needs. Carefully analyze your unit's resources to determine successful partnership strategies based on apparent needs.

Initiate the partnership. Once needs have been cooperatively and carefully identified, the partnership can be pursued. Keep several tips in mind as you move forward. First, narrow the focus of the initiative, but think "big" in terms of the partners' involvement. Many agencies and businesses are eager to collaborate with educational and community-service ventures, especially those projects that involve young people or persons with special needs and that are consistent with their mission. Second, become familiar with the agency you intend to recruit as a partner. Learn about its history, financial position, resource base, and previous involvement in community service and collaboration. Talk with other community members about the agency and its staff. This step is critical if you are to be successful in creating a good first impression and a lasting partnership. Third, identify the principal players within the partner organization. The CEO or president is not always the right person to contact. Often, a separate office exists to deal with community or external relations, and personnel within it will usually make the decisions regarding external partnerships. As you familiarize yourself with potential partners, it will become apparent how to initiate meaningful and timely discussions. Some situations will require an initial phone call, letter, or other type of communication. A simple but meaningful face-to-face meeting is the best way to handle others. Trust your judgment as to what sort of contact fits a given situation, but also determine if an agency has a required protocol for that situation. Before entering serious deliberations with a potential partner, you must also be sure to inform and gain approval from your supervisor. In these times of fiscal restraint, it is difficult to imagine an administrator discouraging collaborative efforts. However, there may be circumstances that you are unaware of that make a specific partnership unappealing or unacceptable to others at your institution (e.g., the timing may not be right, or another unit may be pursuing the same agency).

Once you are sure that there are sufficient common interests between the agency and your unit, and you are comfortable with approaching them with the idea, it is time to bring people to the table to discuss a prospective partnership. In doing so, be sure to extend a personal invitation, provide them with sufficient background materials to read prior to the meeting, and indicate that the purpose of the preliminary discussions is to explore the feasibility of working together to accomplish similar goals. Conduct the meeting in a professional manner. Include a well-defined agenda and a clear proposal for them to review. This proposal should identify the purpose of the initiative, short- and long-term goals, partnership activities, indicators of goal-attainment, constituencies involved, and, most important, the benefits of collaboration for each partner. All involved must see a direct benefit to their respective organizations. Will it provide print and electronic advertising for them? Are there tax breaks or other financial advantages to the partnership? Are the projected outcomes of the partnership directly related to the mission of the agency? Partners will ask or expect you to address these and many other questions. As an administrator, you must anticipate all such questions and be prepared to present realistic answers or suggested solutions.

Capitalize on community assets. After all parties agree that a partnership is desired and could be successful, take inventory of the internal resources available to you. Although you need to maximize the participation of the partners, there may be other community assets that can strengthen the partnership and increase the likelihood of a successful initiative. Combining the assets of two agencies usually results in more than a 1+1 = 2 scenario. Typically, there is a positive ripple effect among other agencies in the community. Think broadly when identifying community agencies and assets that may supplement the specific partnership. Find out about private businesses and city and county governmental agencies that are committed to community needs. Consider the strategic location of the community, the composition of the population, and the successes of past partnerships. Although additional funding in real dollars is always appealing, most community resources will take a different form. For example, consider the use of indoor and outdoor space at no cost, personnel resources, public-relations opportunities, volunteer health services, equipment, supplies, technology, various forms of media services, transportation, and many other potentially costly assets that are essential to the success of community programs. Effective partnerships can link resources for cost savings.

Formalize the partnership. As with any successful and mutually beneficial business arrangement, all partners must be aware of their duties, commitments, and responsibilities. After completing the brainstorming and discussions, formalize the partnership. Be aware that most colleges and universities have a grants and contract office (or other unit with external sponsorship duties) that can assist with this phase. Contact this or a related office at your institution for policies and procedures to follow. As the lead administrator, you should provide a rough-draft document that: describes the partnership; details the goals, objectives, implementation activities, and evaluation of the initiative; stipulates the length of the partnership; explains the financial commitments of all partners; fully discusses the nature of liability; addresses any insurance concerns; speaks to the use of facilities, equipment, and/or personnel; and addresses any other details requiring clarification. This document should receive internal approval before it is released to the external agency. External agencies should be given ample time to review and comment on the agreement or contract. After several drafts, the agreement should be finalized. At this point, it is customary to have the highest-ranking officials of the respective agencies and/or their designees gather for a ceremony highlighting the partnership. Leaders from among the partner organization have an opportunity to publicly acknowledge the intent of the collaborative effort and the value it will bring to the community. This recognition is important for your unit and will bring valuable attention to your efforts. Don't overlook or underestimate this public-relations opportunity.

Encourage collaboration. Not surprisingly, one of the most challenging tasks associated with any partnership is maintaining interest and a high energy level among those working with the initiative on a day-to-day basis. Administrators need to provide leadership and encouragement that sustains the collaborative efforts. You need to be sensitive to this challenge and devote time and energy to fostering support for the partnership among your staff. Within the educational environment, there are a variety of ways to accomplish this. For example, academic administrators can stress the importance of collaborative community-service efforts and reward faculty accordingly within the promotion, retention, and merit processes. Collaborative partnerships naturally complement teaching, scholarship, and service responsibilities and expectations. It is important to help faculty and staff blend their responsibilities with the community partnerships in such a way that they are rewarded for their time and effort. Another way to encourage collaboration is to provide assigned time for faculty to engage in significant partnership activity. In doing so, administrators not only recognize the efforts of the faculty members engaged in the initiative, but also publicly demonstrate the value of the partnership for their unit. Direct or indirect financial remuneration can also be given to faculty for successfully completing such work. Surprisingly, though, some faculty prefer not to receive direct compensation. Instead, many choose to have the equivalent amount of dollars available to them for travel, equipment, or other items that enhance their professional development. Assigning a graduate assistant to a faculty member or partnership program could also prove to be a very motivating factor. Other methods to encourage ongoing collaborative activities include:

- Periodic media events or releases to showcase the partnership and highlight associated individuals. In addition to good public visibility for the partnership, this would provide a forum for recognizing the talents of those professionals who are contributing to the success of the initiative.
- Hosting special open houses and other types of gatherings. This can create additional opportunities to acknowledge those who are responsible for the success of the partnership.
- Presenting highlights and/or results of the partnership at professional conferences and sharing successful methods and procedures with others through various publications.
- Procuring outside funds. Most funding or granting agencies expect collaborative arrangements to serve as problem-solving vehicles. As such, a successful partnership could seek external dollars to support continuation or expansion of its initiative. An external funding agency's recognition of collaborative efforts is very meaningful and usually generates a wealth of positive energy, motivation, and resources for the partnership.

Retain leadership. The success of any partnership depends largely on one partner's sustained leadership. Although the partnership is the result of everyone working together, the future direction of the collaboration is usually determined by an individual's vision and personal efforts. This determination should be the responsibility of the partner with the greatest investment. Investment does not necessarily mean dollars only. It can also refer to time, talent, space, creativity, and derived benefits. Units that initiate partnerships are strategically situated to maintain leadership and to develop a sense of ownership for a successful collaborative venture. In a position of leadership, a unit can capitalize on its efforts by deflecting credit for the successes of the partnership to the collaborators. This generates a wealth of goodwill and clearly identifies the unit as being instrumental in developing the partnership. Administrators should capitalize on their strategic positions to ensure the continued success of partnerships.

Examples of Partnerships

Described below are several examples of HPERD-related partnerships that have been successful for colleges and universities. Many factors that led to the success of these collaborative efforts were unique to the particular institutions involved and may not be present in your situation. As described above, each unit needs to examine how its strengths, goals, and resources best fit local circumstances. Experienced administrators advise that units should be ready for expansion, since successful partnerships breed more activity. New projects will develop as offshoots of others and other external agencies will want to be part of the action.

Partnership between a college of HPER and a city police department. This partnership evolved from a university program funded by the National Collegiate Athletic Association and the U.S. Department of Health and Human Services. The university's National Youth Sports Program (NYSP) grant provides funds to implement a comprehensive educational enrichment program for youths (ages 10 to 16) from low-income families. Included in its programming are alcohol and drug education, health education, gang and violence prevention, and many other elements. Within the same community, a police department was attempting to develop a summer program to supplement their school-year Drug Abuse Resistance Education (DARE) and Gang Resistance Education and Training (GREAT) efforts. Leaders from each organization became aware of the duplication potential of their programs and met to discuss each other's goals, needs, and partnership prospects. The resulting partnership has flourished. The College of HPER has benefited by having several police officers on staff at no cost to the program. The police department provides an AOD specialist and other staff to NYSP as well. In addition, the program receives transportation and other supplemental funds available only to the police department. The benefits of the partnership extend far beyond the funding, though. The effects on public relations have been outstanding. University and police department staff members have presented the success of the partnership at conferences. In addition, the program has been successful at procuring external funds from sources such as the county health department, the area community foundation, a university foundation, and other area agencies.

Partnership between a PK-12 public school district and a university to fund a grant-proposal writer. The procurement of funds through various granting agencies can enhance programs of all types. This need exists at all levels of education. Recognizing this need led to a very productive partnership between a university and a PK-12 school district. After much discussion, an agreement was struck to jointly fund a grant-proposal writer. Proposals are limited to those projects that will benefit both the university teacher-education programs and the school district. A committee composed of district and university staff screens potential projects. This partnership has been an overwhelming success both financially and programmatically. Many faculty members who have not been involved in grantseeking or PK-12 relations have used this partnership as a steppingstone to desired collaborative activity. In addition to the grants that assist each partner, the collaboration has led to many more cooperative ventures. Most of these positive relations would not have occurred without the proposal-writer partnership being in place.

Partnership between a university-based cardiac rehabilitation program and a local hospital. Many universities can provide resources to community agencies in the form of students, facilities, expertise, and services. One such partnership was developed to provide university-based cardiac rehabilitation services to Phase III postoperative patients. The local community had a need for a facility and staff. The local hospital provides funding for a staff member to coordinate services between the hospital and university. Many benefits result for each partner. The university's students are provided with necessary clinical experiences, a graduate student is funded, patients are available to serve as potential subjects for student and faculty research, and many positive public relations are garnered from the effort. The hospital is able to monitor its patients closely, use a low-cost facility, and access the expertise of many faculty, all without the full cost of an in-house cardiac rehabilitation program.

Graduate assistantships to teach elementary physical education. A common higher education partnership in many communities involves the funding of graduate assistants to provide various types of professional services. One example of this is contracting or partnering with local elementary schools to provide instructional services. Both parties benefit from this relationship. The university is able to fund a student, the school often serves as a clinical education site and a demonstration site for various activities, and subjects are available for research. The school benefits from professional services at an often-reduced cost (compared to a regularly employed teacher). The relationship will also often result in the presence of many college students to assist with tutoring and other needed services in the partnership school. Another common component of this type of relationship involves giving a schoolteacher release time from the K-12 role to work in the higher education setting. Preservice teacher-education programs are greatly enhanced by the presence of a veteran teacher sharing experiences and suggestions.

Partnership between a long-term care facility and a university department of recreation management and therapeutic recreation. A local facility that provides services to persons with Alzheimer's disease (AD) was a common site for university therapeutic-recreation clinical students. This partnership exposed students to clients and provided faculty with information about a private foundation that funds projects for AD. The partnership was expanded through the submission of a proposal to this foundation that was funded for approximately $85,000. Without the initial partnership, this grant project would not have evolved. Results included community service, research studies, teaching improvement due to real-world clinical experiences, and scholarship through publications and presentations.

Making Partnerships Work

Responsibility for sustaining the enthusiasm and momentum of partnerships will often fall to academic administrators. Plan for this as the partnership is being implemented, and be prepared for a predictable lull after a certain time period. Of course, the degree of the partnership's success will dictate how much effort is required to maintain interest.

Several suggestions for maintaining partnerships can be culled from past successful ventures. A planned review of each partner's goals and vision should take place on a regular basis, since agencies often change their focus or reevaluate their mission. Another key element is having the right individuals in leadership roles. These key players are often not administrators. Experience will be an important factor as you select personnel to lead and sustain collaborative efforts with external agencies. Not all faculty and staff will want to pursue this type of activity, nor will they have the skills, temperament, and knowledge to lead partnerships. Keeping new staff members involved in partnerships is a good way to avoid burnout among the veteran participants. New personnel should become involved so that they understand the importance of these external activities to the overall mission of their unit.

Successful partnerships will lead to other opportunities with the same or other agencies. Be prepared for these offshoot projects; as previously mentioned, however, you should be cautious about overextending your time, effort, and resources. Stay focused on what your unit is trying to accomplish. Don't get sidetracked and "lose" faculty to outside initiatives—it can happen fast! Keep ahead of the trends and project possible scenarios before they become real problems.

Evaluating the progress of a partnership is necessary to determine if continuation is warranted. A series of questions developed by Clark and Lacey (1997) can help administrators assess if partnership progress is sufficient and acceptable. These assessment questions should be modified to meet the specific circumstances of your partnership, and both partners should be involved in this evaluation.

- Have the short-term objectives been achieved? Is there progress? Why/why not?
- Does the partner understand the content of the partnership work (the what and why)? What evidence is there of this understanding?
- Does the partner understand the process of the work (the how)? What evidence is there?
- Does the partner "walk the talk"? What evidence is there?
- What are the strengths of the partnership?
- Does the partner attend to the totality of the partnership framework?
- Does the partner make a contribution to your agency's strategic interests? How?
- Is there expansion (actual or planned) of the number of individuals, groups, and organizations involved in the partnership?
- What have been the most significant successes of the partnership to date?
- What have been the most persistent problems for the partnership to date?

These and other assessment questions should be part of the evaluation component for partnerships. Planning systematic evaluation should be part of your initial partnership agreement. Take time to implement the evaluation, share the results, and use the information to improve your decision-making. Evaluation data will be an expectation of other funding agencies and a necessary source of information for future planning.

Administrators play a key role in the development, implementation, and evaluation of partnerships. These collaborative relations can provide opportunities for many positive outcomes. However, leaders must be aware that not all ideas will yield positive results. Ramaley (2000) provides several important lessons regarding partnerships that apply to HPERD areas and offer valuable insight for administrators:

- Each partnership has unique elements shaped by history, capacity, cultures, missions, expectations, and challenges faced by each participating group. It is not easy to work across multiple organizational cultures and communication patterns.

- Any partnership must be based on the academic strengths and philosophy of the campus. An ideal partnership will match institutional strengths with the assets and interests of the community.
- To ease the problem of multiple organizational cultures, the needs and capacities of the community (rather than the prerogatives and assumptions of higher education) must define the approach that the university takes to forming a partnership.
- There is no such thing as a universal "community," nor are there usually agreed-upon spokespersons for any community you choose to embrace. Often, partnerships are fragmented by competing interests within the community, on campus, or both.
- It takes time to understand what elements make up a particular community and how people experience their membership in the community.
- Some communities are being "partnered" to the point of exhaustion. It is often necessary to help community organizations and smaller agencies become capable of serving as effective partners.
- In some smaller communities, there may not be enough volunteer or not-for-profit activities to absorb the energies of a college or university interested in full engagement. In such cases, the campus may need to create, in cooperation with its neighbors, the infrastructure necessary to sustain community-based work.
- The early rush of enthusiasm can be replaced by fatigue and burnout unless the partners identify and recruit additional talent early on, from both on and off campus.
- It is important to establish a strong commitment to a "culture of evidence" that traces the progress of a project or a collaboration as it develops, not just at the end. The lessons learned from continuous evaluation can sustain the work and allow it to grow to a scale that can make a genuine difference in the community. Involve students in the integral part of the work of collaboration so that they learn skills of communication, problem-solving, and shared learning early.

Administrators and others preparing to venture forth with partnerships should carefully study the experiences of others. Seek the advice of other administrators who have been active in community partnerships. The benefits reaped through careful planning and continued assessment will be worth the investment.

Summary

As colleges and universities continue to enhance and expand their services and impact, they must become better partners with community constituencies. Partnerships offer an effective and convenient means to remain in touch with the community and enhance the resource base of all involved. Effective sharing of personnel and other resources between PK-12 schools, higher-education institutions, public and private agencies, and businesses can maximize efforts to achieve shared goals and visions. Administrators play a key role in establishing community partnerships; they must take the lead to form collaborative relations and a "real" presence in the community. Planning must take place to ensure that partnerships will achieve their intended goals and not drain resources. Use the power of partnerships to help you and your unit achieve your goals and vision.

About the Author

Garth Tymeson is a professor in, and interim dean of, the College of Health, Physical Education, Recreation, and Teacher Education at the University of Wisconsin–La Crosse. Previously, he served as associate dean and director of university graduate studies for this institution, and as an associate professor at Northern Illinois University.

References

Clark, T., & Lacey, R. (1997). *Learning by doing: Panasonic partnerships and systematic school reform.* Delray Beach, FL: St. Lucie Press.

Hastad, D., & Tymeson, G. (1997). Demonstrating visionary leadership through community partnerships. *Journal of Physical Education, Recreation & Dance, 68*(5), 47-50.

O'Sullivan, M., Tannehill, D., Knop, N., Pope, C., & Henninger, M. (1999). A school-university collaborative journey through relevance and meaning in an urban high school physical education program. *Quest, 51*(3), 225-243.

Ramaley, J. (2000). Embracing civic responsibility. *AAHE Bulletin, 52*(7), 9-11.

Stoel, C., Togneri, W., & Brown, P. (1992). *What works: School/college partnerships to improve poor and minority student achievement.* Washington, DC: American Association for Higher Education.

Wilbur, F., & Lambert, L. (1995). *Linking America's schools and colleges: Guide to partnerships and national directory.* Jaffrey, NH: Anker.

20 Establishing Business Relationships within the Community

Richard C. Miller, *Dean, School of Health Sciences and Human Performance, Ithaca College*

You have to have patience and good communication skills.

— Don McKillip

One of the many challenges confronting colleges and universities today is the need to solicit and secure funding beyond those resources acquired through tuition and fees. While many research institutions have at their disposal dedicated professionals who possess grant-writing and fundraising expertise, they remain the exceptions to the rule within higher education. Seeking creative means to secure external resources remains a major challenge for many institutions.

Today, employers are concerned about the quality of the future workforce and the preparation of students to meet higher standards of achievement in a variety of professional fields. Employers look for opportunities to build a qualified workforce by offering potential employees internships, cooperative education, part-time work, and shadowing opportunities. To achieve these outcomes, collaboration with educational institutions is deemed essential.

Establishing Relationships

Establishing a mutually beneficial working relationship between higher education and the local business community ensures economic prosperity in the community, enhances understanding between the partners, raises the level of motivation and educational achievement, and provides students, faculty, and local-business employees with access to better equipment. In addition, such a relationship ensures that today's businesses and students are equipped with the skills they need for tomorrow, and that community concerns are adequately addressed.

Many businesses tend to focus on two primary educational reforms—moving to higher educational standards and school-to-work initiatives. These efforts must be linked, and the role of the employer is critical in making them successful. Whether our young people go to college or directly into the workforce, the required core skills are the same—academic achievement, problem-solving skills, and the ability to learn, communicate, and effectively apply interpersonal and group skills. Without these skills, they will not find successful careers, and employers will not have the high-quality personnel needed to compete in the global marketplace.

Within the disciplines of health, physical education, and recreation (HPER), administrators and faculty have begun to expand their search for additional resource support by seeking mutually beneficial relationships within their local business communities. In order to maintain program viability in the face of tightening budgets and stagnant enrollments, administrators must continue to employ management strategies that foster such relationships.

As educational institutions commit themselves to the professional preparation of future business employees, business leaders understandably have a vested interest in the quality and health status of these prospective workers. Recognizing that the business community must invest heavily in the professional development of its workforce, many employers tend to respond positively to educational programs that place emphasis on health. Such is the case with businesses that support corporate fitness programs, structured leisure activities, and relaxation and stress-relief programs. Colleges and universities with educational programs in these areas would profit from establishing partnerships with these businesses.

Community as Resource

Most colleges and universities have never been able to acquire sufficient resources to meet all the needs of their existing educational programs. Private giving by individuals, foundations, and industries, which had long provided operating and capital funds for private institutions, has become increasingly important for public colleges and universities as well, not merely as budget relief, but as an important source of core support. While relying on resource support from foundations and individuals, college and university administrators and faculty would be well advised to focus their attention on establishing partnerships with the business community to assist in bearing the financial burden faced as result of dwindling funds.

Identifying resource strategies that HPER disciplines can use to attract the interest of the business community should be a shared responsibility between faculty and administrators, involving both tactical and strategic planning initiatives. Business executives respond positively when planned partnerships with health-related programs have clearly stated objectives and evaluative criteria that can lead to operational efficiency and greater productivity from the workforce.

University as Resource

Healthcare in the 1990s has undergone significant changes. Not only have health and disease-management programs been established through hospital-based initiatives, but recent movements toward medically oriented fitness/wellness programs have offered new and challenging opportunities for clinical exercise physiologists from kinesiology departments housed in institutions of higher education. For example, an exercise-science or cardiac-rehabilitation program could help a business establish a corporate-fitness or disease-management program that could include health and fitness assessments of employees, smoking-cessation programs, nutrition- and drug-education programs, and stress-management programs, all of which would lead to a healthier and more productive workforce. In turn, businesses may be inclined to invest in those educational programs that are preparing future professionals who, as prospective employees, would already be trained to sustain the established corporate programs.

The disturbing trend of increasingly higher incidents of drug and alcohol abuse among teens and young adults gives rise to serious health-related consequences and places greater stress on an already burdened health-care industry. Substance abuse among this statistically at-risk population creates opportunities for health-related education programs, health-maintenance organizations (HMOs), and hospitals to become more closely associated. Many HMOs that provide substance-abuse treatment benefits to their members may be inclined to fund such education programs if they are provided by institutions of higher education. Health-education programs within HPER units are ideal candidates to establish business relationships with local and regional HMOs and hospitals.

It is important, however, that HPER administrators and faculty recognize and understand the important differences between profit-oriented businesses and academic institutions in planning objectives and evaluating outcomes. Typically, academic objectives are multifaceted and ambiguous, and disagreements can arise about the most appropriate criteria with which to assess the attainment of these objectives. Businesses measure achievement during a given period of time based on factors such as net profit, rate of return, and change in market share. Given this difference, HPER administrators and faculty must relate the outcomes of having a healthy workforce to these measures of business success and productivity.

Another potential initiative between HPER and the business community could involve the assessment of the work capacity of employees injured on the job. Professionals in the fields of kinesiology, biomechanics, and movement education could establish assessment teams to evaluate the functional capabilities of injured employees (those on Worker's Compensation) during and following their prescribed therapies. These assessment protocols would provide valuable information to business executives as to the preparedness of injured workers to re-enter the workforce. Business executives would be more inclined to invest their resources in programs that provide such valuable services.

Many academic institutions are located in communities where architectural and construction businesses are likely to be awarded contracts for the planning and construction of campus facilities. It is not uncommon for a single firm to work on multiple facilities for HPER and athletic programs. These frequent business relationships can provide mutually beneficial outcomes for all involved. The construction and architectural industries place strong emphasis on high-quality work in the hopes of attracting repeat clients. In many cases, these continuing relationships result in considerable cost savings for the academic institution, in addition to the possibility of combining the shared expertise of industry and college personnel in addressing problems and concerns relative to facility planning and maintenance. Furthermore, architectural and construction executives are frequently seen showcasing their work on a campus to other potential clients; a strong business relationship between institutions of higher education and the architectural and construction industries serves to focus attention on high-quality planning and construction.

Recent developments in the formation of private ventures by institutions of higher education can be tailored to provide educational services to companies. In July 2000, Duke University's business school established Duke Corporate Education, Inc., to meet the needs of the business community for courses in leadership development, strategic planning, and marketing operations. These and similar ventures with the business community can provide for a shareholder interest by the educational corporation with remaining stock being divided between private investors and employees. While such ventures may seem too speculative for many institutions, the provision of educational services to the business community may result in long-term financial gains that are mutually beneficial.

Exercise- and health-science programs in a number of institutions have formed solid business relationships with local governments through the establishment of wellness and fitness centers that provide health and fitness assessment of employees such as firemen and policemen. These programs serve to cement "town and gown" relationships that have far-reaching benefits. In addition, faculty can serve as consultants to the business community in planning new programs and recommending cost-effective measures to maximize employee productivity and improve job satisfaction.

Research and Training

The future clearly belongs to those communities in which it is recognized that a modern workforce must rely on research and training that only higher-education institutions can provide. Administrators in all professional fields, including HPER, must present a clearly articulated vision of higher education's contributions to the well-being of the nation and its citizenry. Furthermore, today's markets, including the healthcare market, stretch around the world. If business and government leaders accept the view that the health of any democratic society is inextricably tied to the health of its citizens, then HPER disciplines should seize the opportunity to articulate their contribution to the overall well-being of all citizens.

Business leaders increasingly value international experiences in the graduates they hire. Students in HPER disciplines who have international experiences represent a cadre of well-educated leaders who will help create a positive international business and political climate. Establishing relationships with multinational businesses can lead to steady, non-politicized support for institutional research and development.

While institutions of higher education look to the business community for funding support of mutually beneficial endeavors, one of the most recent growth areas in business and management over the past decade has been entrepreneurism. Few examples exist within HPER programs of collaborative efforts with the business community to encourage intellectual entrepreneurship. Given the business industry's considerable experience in identifying the qualities of a successful entrepreneur, a relationship between higher education and business could encourage faculty to think outside of disciplinary boundaries and take calculated and institutionally supported risks. Academic administrators of HPER programs should seek solutions to problems through the study of the organizational culture of successful businesses while exploring non-traditional models. Educational programs can benefit from association with successful businesses whose core ideology is not based solely on profit. Establishing such partnerships will be an inviting challenge as we progress through the 21st century.

Engaging the local business community in a dialogue on common interests and concerns is a reasonably uncomplicated process. Most local businesses and institutions of higher education contribute significantly to local economies and to the quality of life enjoyed by citizens. If businesses and universities accept the view that they share common values and a commitment to the well-being of their stakeholders, then common ground clearly exists for a meaningful dialogue. Another area that business and higher education have explored is information management and the problems associated with how to handle too much information. With a more knowledgeable workforce and increasing demand for educational opportunities for employees, colleges and universities are collaborating with local businesses to establish distance-learning programs using educational technology and technical support from both sectors. HPER units are ideally situated to take advantage of these opportunities. For example, a sports-nutrition professor could teach high school athletes, coaches, and parents who are located far away from the campus about proper eating habits and dietary supplements using equipment purchased by a local nutrition business or restaurant consortium.

Athletic departments have had longstanding relationships with soft-drink manufacturers and other companies. These businesses have purchased scoreboards, equipment, and other items in return for the opportunity to advertise their products. Although some criticism has been directed at these types of relationships, many have resulted in sustained, long-term program support. Still, administrators have too often been focused on the financial advantages of these business relationships while giving the social and ethical implications secondary consideration. Clearly, a proper balance needs to be encouraged, and both faculty and student input should be solicited.

With demographic data suggesting that teacher shortages are imminent in a variety of areas, university teacher-education programs need to assist businesses that have employees who want to share their skills and experiences in today's classrooms. Work-based learning strategies and initiatives can be funded by businesses and conducted in university classrooms. This presents a unique opportunity for HPER disciplines, since professionals in these fields compose a large share of the teaching pool. With a focus on wellness, fitness, and healthy living practices in the public schools, the cost of continuing-education programs for business employees with an interest in these areas is likely to be subsidized by their employers.

Business executives consider it very advantageous to have their employees contribute to the community. Employees often become involved in local sports programs for youths (e.g., as volunteer coaches). Many HPER programs have long concentrated on preparing students and adults to coach youth sports, and local businesses demonstrate their contribution to the community by sponsoring such programs. Therefore, the opportunity for HPER programs to establish a relationship with the business community clearly exists. Businesses could be solicited to support coaching seminars, workshops, and conferences in which educators and intercollegiate athletics coaches provide the instruction.

Seeking
Shared Values

Similarly, local soft-drink companies, hospitals, and medical centers can sponsor educational programs on dietary supplements, diet and nutrition for athletes, injury prevention, and targeted training protocols. A committed collaborative effort involving business and higher education providing a service in these areas would not only be mutually beneficial to the partners, but also lead to a safer environment for competitive youth sports.

Summary

In summary, combining the strengths and resources of local businesses with those of higher education can result in the following benefits:

- greater potential for a more highly skilled and productive workforce;
- more opportunities for the increased marketability of college students who benefit from hands-on experiences;
- enhanced ability of business employees and college faculty to apply their skills and talents within and outside their respective work environments;
- increased service to the local community; and
- a sense of satisfaction in reaching mutually defined goals and objectives.

Establishing business relationships within the community not only provides mutually beneficial outcomes for the participating organizations, but also contributes to the health, well-being, and quality of life of all citizens

About the Author

Richard C. Miller, dean of the School of Health Sciences and Human Performance at Ithaca College, has an exercise-science background and has been involved in higher-education administration for 24 years.

SECTION V

Closure

21 Vision: Requisite for Success

Thomas J. Templin, ***Professor and Head, Department of Health, Kinesiology, and Leisure Studies, Purdue University***

B. Don Franks, ***Professor, Department of Kinesiology, University of Maryland***

Prizes aren't awarded for predicting rain, but for building arks.

Thomas J. Templin

In his book about leadership, Perkins (2000) used the fascinating adventure of Sir Ernest Shakelton as an illustration of what it takes to lead a group on any journey—particularly one riddled with constant challenge. In 1914, a British expedition led by Shakelton set sail on the ship *Endurance* with the goal of reaching Antarctica and achieving the first overland crossing of this frozen continent. As Perkins (2000) described it:

> *Shakelton had a clear vision and a plan for how to achieve it. Shakelton intended to sail from London to Buenos Aires and then to the island of South Georgia. From South Georgia, the expedition would enter the Weddell Sea, cross Antarctica, and exit on the other side, where the ship would be waiting. Having calculated the times and distances, Shakelton believed the transcontinental journey could be completed in 120 days. (p. 2)*

Even with a handpicked crew and the Latin motto "Fortitudine Vincimus" ("by endurance we conquer") as his guiding light, Shakelton's journey didn't work out quite as he had planned. At one point, the vessel became trapped in ice. It was then that Shakelton's real leadership abilities and the fortitude, courage, and survival skills of his crew were put to test under the most severe conditions (remember that the coldest temperature ever recorded in Antarctica was a mere minus 128.6 degrees Fahrenheit!).

While the crew waited for the ship to be magically released from the grip of the ice, the ever-crushing blows of the frozen sea eventually opened the vessel like a tin can. The crew was forced to abandon it and set off over ice floes, dragging life-rafts and supplies along with the slimmest hope of survival. As their supplies dwindled and hopes faded, the men eventually had to set off in their life-rafts on the open sea when the ice pack opened. Miraculously, the rafts drifted to Elephant Island after 497 days, where the men recuperated while Shakelton plotted out the next plan of survival—namely, for him and five others to set course in the best of the rafts with the hope of reaching South Georgia. After 16 horrendous days, Shakelton and his five mates made it to South Georgia; however, they were on the wrong side of the island, the one that was covered with "treacherous" glaciers.

Shakelton and his two "best able" men then set out to reach a whaling station, and after enduring four dangerous days on foot, they made it to safety. This was followed by the rescue of the three men left on the other side of the island, eventually ending with the subsequent rescue of those left on Elephant Island, 634 days after they had originally set sail from South Georgia! The last rescue took four attempts, all led by Shakelton. He had not forgotten his crew and his role as their leader.

While his methods may have been extreme, in that they led to unnecessary risk, they did demonstrate how an individual's vision can lead others through the severest of tests. They also highlighted his ability to deal with unexpected events that changed not only his immediate goals and plans, but also his vision itself. Perkins (2000) gives countless examples of how Shakelton coped with hardship, conflict, and sinking morale to bolster his crew and motivate them to take responsibility and survive. He uses this amazing adventure as an example of the leadership qualities needed to achieve success:

1. Never lose sight of the ultimate goal, and focus energy on short-term objectives.
2. Set a personal example with visible, memorable symbols and behaviors.
3. Instill optimism and self-confidence, but stay grounded in reality.
4. Take care of yourself: maintain your stamina and let go of guilt.
5. Reinforce the team message constantly: "We are one—we live or die together."
6. Minimize status differences and insist on courtesy and mutual respect.
7. Master conflict—deal with anger in small doses, engage dissidents, and avoid needless power struggles.
8. Find something to celebrate and something to laugh about.
9. Be willing to take the "Big Risk."
10. Never give up—there's always another move.

From Perkins (2000)

While this recitation of Shakelton's story is not intended to suggest that survival is the "vision" to be cherished and pursued in health, kinesiology, and leisure studies (HKLS) (although we know that survival is a real issue in some universities and colleges), this chapter will reinforce some of the above principles as we address the concepts of vision, community, empowerment, quality, and commitment. Anyone sitting in the administrator's chair within a HKLS school or department must possess various leadership qualities if the unit is to succeed. As with Shakelton, there will be times when you must lead on the edge.

While Shakelton's ultimate goal was the overland crossing of Antarctica, this vision was quickly redefined to one of basic survival—a vision wrought with uncertainty. Yet this uncertainty also required decisive action and the involvement of others in plotting a shared course of survival. Similarly, both vision and action are needed for any group or organization to progress. Nanus (1992) defined vision as

> ....a realistic, credible, attractive future for your organization. It is your articulation of a destination toward which your organization should aim, a future that in important ways is better, more successful, or more desirable for your organization than is the present....Vision always deals with the future. Indeed, vision is where tomorrow begins, for it expresses what you and others who share the vision will be working hard to create....

> ....[T]he right vision attracts commitment and energizes people, creates meaning in workers' lives, establishes a standard of excellence, bridges the present and the future, transcends the status quo, and provides an indispensable guide to what must be preserved and what can be cut back with least risk to future viability. (pp. 8, 16-18)

The key result of establishing the "right vision" is empowerment: that is, empowering others who share the vision to act in a way that is valued and legitimized by colleagues. Belasco (1990) stated that "vision empowers people to change" and that an "empowering vision spells out clearly what you want and inspires people to produce it. A vision specifies a mutual destination—the place everyone agrees to go—and the major activities to get you there" (p. 98).

Within and across our disciplines, this question of vision is under constant scrutiny. What visions are held within the HKLS communities? What do our visions focus on: research, curricula, teaching, service, administrative structure and function, or fundraising? Must these visions be shared by all within the academy? Are different visions, missions, and structures appropriate for different types of institutions? Numerous treatises have been written on the future of our fields and on the appropriate vision, mission, purposes, structures, and strategies for promoting a new HKLS within the academy (Wilmore, 1998; Kretchmar, 1999). Clearly, debates and arguments will persist about whether we should emphasize research, preparation of applied practitioners, or service provision, but we must not be consumed by such debates. Can we not establish a vision that recognizes the importance of each activity to the promotion of our profession? Can we not work toward integration of research, teaching, and service? Certainly, different individuals and institutions will have different priorities for each area, depending on their context, but it is here where administrators and faculty must discuss the value of shared vision and compromise to reach that vision.

Vision in HKLS

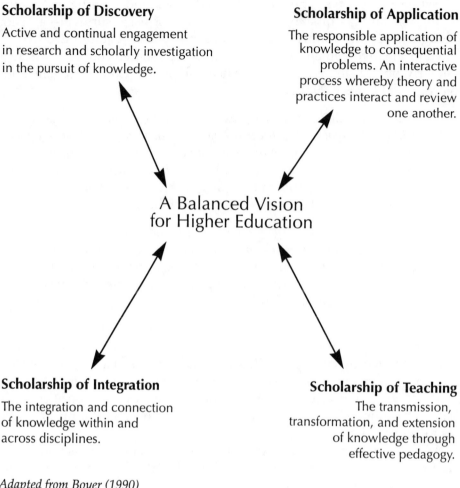

FIGURE 21.1
Boyer's
Balanced Vision
for Higher Education

Scholarship of Discovery

Active and continual engagement in research and scholarly investigation in the pursuit of knowledge.

Scholarship of Application

The responsible application of knowledge to consequential problems. An interactive process whereby theory and practices interact and review one another.

A Balanced Vision for Higher Education

Scholarship of Integration

The integration and connection of knowledge within and across disciplines.

Scholarship of Teaching

The transmission, transformation, and extension of knowledge through effective pedagogy.

Adapted from Boyer (1990)

Boyer's (1990) pioneering vision promotes a balanced view of the scholarship of discovery, integration, application, and teaching that is closely connected to this perspective (figure 21.1). As Boyer stated,

> ....the most important obligation now confronting the nation's colleges and universities is to break out of the tired old teaching versus research debate and define, in more creative ways, what it means to be a scholar. It's time to recognize the full range of faculty talent and the great diversity of functions [that] higher education must perform. (p. xii)

This does not dismiss the importance of high-quality performance, but it does stress the acceptance of a wide range of priorities and roles within the academy. Six reports from the Kellogg Commission on the Future of State and Land-Grant Universities (1997, 1998a,b, 1999, 2000a,b) reinforced, extended, and presented examples of Boyer's model at various colleges and universities. Combined, these reports provide an excellent vision for the future of higher education.

As one "audits" an existing vision or considers the development of a new vision for a school or department, various questions may be of help (Nanus, 1992):

- What is the current mission or purpose of the school or department?
- What values does the school or department provide to society? Is it engaged?
- What is the institutional framework within which the school or department operates?
- What is the school or department's unique position within the university?
- What does it take to be successful?
- What are the current values, principles, and the culture that govern behavior and decision-making?
- What are the strengths and weaknesses of the organization, and how can strengths be maintained and weaknesses eliminated or reduced?
- What is the organization's current operating structure and strategy?
- If the organization stays on its current path, where will it be headed in the next decade?
- Does the school/university leadership agree with this direction?

The answers to these questions are linked to the structural context of a department, school, or university and will influence the scope and direction of each. Ultimately, these answers lead to a shared commitment and understanding within a department or school. For example, the kinesiology faculty at the University of Colorado–Boulder engaged in a change process whereby the vision of the department is now focused on the study of physical activity, disease prevention, and aging. As Moore (1998) described it, "our curriculum continues to evolve to reflect this theme and provides a logical and timely link to changes in national healthcare and research policies to the extent that the importance of physical activity in disease prevention and the promotion of successful aging have been clearly and unequivocally acknowledged" (p. 201). This vision has been operationalized through shared research and teaching missions within the department and through interdisciplinary connections with other university partners. This department has created a vision and acted on it, and is on a pathway that will lead to many successful years ahead.

Naturally, there are many pathways to follow; again, context plays a major role in the development of a unit's vision. For example, some institutions (e.g., the University of Maryland) have chosen to include programs in exercise science, behavioral science, pedagogy, and the social-cultural aspects of physical activity in one department, while other institutions (e.g., Florida State University, the University of South Carolina) have separated exercise science from physical education. Some HKLS-related units are in a college of arts and sciences (e.g., at Arizona State University), a school of liberal arts (e.g., at Purdue University), or a college of education (e.g., at Ohio State University). Some units are in traditional HKLS contexts and may include dance, physical therapy, or other departments (e.g., at Indiana University, East Carolina University, the University of Wisconsin). Each can lend a unique vision to the future and make contributions to the goals listed in Boyer and the Kellogg Commission reports.

Finally, one must attempt to characterize the personal vision of a unit's leader. The PEW Foundation (PEW Higher Education Round Table, 1996) stated that "a very good chair can be said to possess both vertical and outside vision of the discipline and horizontal and insider vision of the institution" (p. 6). Perhaps the greatest criticism that we have observed in evaluations of a deans or chairs centers on one's lack of vision and one's inability to address and articulate a vision with others. Oftentimes, it is difficult or impossible to discern whether or not an individual leader has stated, suggested, or recommended a particular vision for an organization. Certainly, standard mission statements abound throughout our universities and colleges. Normative statements related to the promotion of a healthier society through research, teaching, and service, or to the promotion of a high-quality unit through the recruitment of outstanding faculty, staff, and students, are not surprising to anyone. The problem is that such statements don't often inspire or provoke shared values or action. We all want a healthier society and outstanding people within our organizations, but are there other visions and principles beyond these admirable notions that can be shared and acted upon be others? Can a leader develop and promote a balanced vision?

Community Building, Empowerment, and Quality

Of course, having a vision or set of visions isn't enough. The success of any program within the academy calls for many things, but three ingredients that are particularly important are (1) a sense of community among the program's members, (2) their sense of authority over the program's actions and future, and (3) a strong and observable commitment to quality within the program. An organization's vision, sense of mission, and objectives will be difficult to achieve without these characteristics. Without community-building, there is no shared vision. Without empowerment, there is no commitment to a vision. Without quality, there is no attainable vision. Below, we will address each concept briefly.

Community, Empowerment, and Teams

Templin (2000) referred to the work of Peck (1987), who addressed the need for community in any organization: "Peck writes that the seeds of community reside in humanity, which is characterized by inclusiveness, commitment, consensus, realism, contemplation, a safe place to work, a group that can fight gracefully, a group that has spirit, and [most] important, a group [that] takes on varied leadership roles" (p. 12). This suggests that administrators, faculty, staff, and students should work together in a supportive culture wherein decisions are mutually agreed upon, where there is frequent interaction with members of the community, and where there is trust, mutual respect, and toleration of differences, generational or otherwise. Peck calls this a "group of all leaders." In such a community, people are empowered based on their respect for these principles and for one another, and on their ability to contribute to the community in varied ways.

It is when these principles are aligned with the vision and mission of an organization that people are empowered to take actions that advance the unit. The fact that such action will be productive, valued, and considered legitimate should be understood by leaders not as a threat to their leadership, but as a support system for it. People want to be perceived as valued members of a community who can participate in and influence decisions. Hence, the leader of today needs to "let go" and involve others in those decisions that influence the future of the organization, even if it means experiencing and tolerating failure from time to time. Locking others out of such decisions is an affront to one's colleagues and will reduce any sense of community that a unit is able to establish.

How does one go about fostering a sense of belonging and participation? The key to empowerment is delegation and team-building. Delegation centers on empowering others to take on leadership roles in the conduct of a task or the solution of a problem. There are very talented people in every school and department, and it is important to solicit their involvement. The leader must trust, be committed to, and believe in the talents of others in the delegation of various roles (e.g., associate and assistant deans, graduate and undergraduate directors, development officers, academic advisors, fitness directors, lab directors). Delegation must be real, not superficial; soliciting participation in menial tasks will not build community or belief in a leader. Leaders cannot delegate and share responsibility while at the same time looking over their colleagues' shoulders and scrutinizing each and every action or decision. If disagreement results, the leader must find a way to address an issue without subverting the delegation process. By so doing, the leader's integrity will be reinforced (i.e., delegation will be viewed as genuine). Of course, accountability is a close friend of delegation. Those who have been charged to lead various areas are accountable to bring about positive processes and results within a school or department. Delegation also allows unit members to express and demonstrate their commitment. Are they willing to take on additional roles? Are they willing to sacrifice their time, energy, and personal progress on behalf of others? Service in these roles brings on great responsibility, and it should be commended and rewarded.

Delegation through the creation of teams that have a project orientation will foster a sense of community and empowerment as well. But team-making has certain important characteristics that one should keep in mind. Katzenbach and Smith (1993) advocated teamwork and defined a team as "a small number of people with complementary skills who are committed to a common purpose, set of performance goals, and approach for which they hold themselves mutually accountable" (p. 112). The words "team" and "teamwork" should never represent platitudes, but rather a set of people working together with a sense of purpose and desired outcomes, agreed-upon work and meeting processes, reflection and study, open communication, commitment, individual and collective accountability, and support for one another. Typically, teams bring recommendations to a larger body for consideration, but in some cases, teams may be charged as representatives of the school or department to produce something (e.g., an annual report or guidelines for laboratory use) or to make decisions (e.g., concerning admissions). The use of teams has been very beneficial at the lead author's department (see Templin, 2000) in relation to a variety of recommendations brought to the entire faculty (e.g., teams addressing curriculum, graduate programs, interdisciplinary linkages, facilities, funding, administration, marketing, service programs). Building and monitoring team performance is critical; thus the reader is referred to Katzenbach and Smith (1993) for a set of guidelines to consider.

Bringing your unit together from time to time beyond regularly scheduled school or department meetings to revisit, evaluate, discuss, or develop collective vision, mission, objectives, plans, and tasks is an important part of community-building. Having a time to share impressions of how the "team" is doing as a collective body sends a strong message that the leader cares about how others are feeling and moves the leader beyond the routine management tasks that seem to occupy much of an administrator's life today. At times, these meetings will be critical to activities centering on major change. As pointed out in Templin (2000) and Wilmore (1998), collective assessment and planning activities are critical to the change process and to the maintenance of existing programs (Reekie & Wilkinson, 1997). This is difficult and very time consuming work, but it is essential to a unit's growth and to the realization of its vision.

Finally, it is important to invite one's superiors (e.g., a dean) to informally discuss vision, events, issues, or challenges in the school or department. As in most "families," it is important to touch base from time to time. Not doing so breeds isolation and a sense that no one seems to care about an individual member of the family (school or department). You never know what good may result from such sharing. Most difficulties today result from misinformation or misunderstanding between people. Why not create a forum where people can come together to gain a better understanding of an individual's or unit's vision and discuss ways of fulfilling these goals? It just might lead to increased support and resources to meet these ends.

Quality

Without high-quality group members dedicated to high-quality performance, a vision will be impossible to achieve. Quality is expected on every front within and outside of higher education. No one walks around espousing how wonderful it is to pursue mediocrity. Professional journals don't solicit mediocre contributions from authors. University presidents, deans, and department chairs don't send out annual reports addressing the mediocre year they have just experienced. To the contrary, we are always stressing the pursuit of excellence in every aspect of our research, teaching, and service efforts. Administrators, students, parents, the public, and legislators all expect quality. Quality determines the future of schools and departments and of those individuals who work in them. Lack of quality can at times bring about devastating outcomes.

Yet the definition of quality may depend on the context or set of people to which the term is applied. There is ample evidence of this within the academy in relation to departmental survival, promotion reviews, funding decisions, faculty and student recruitment decisions, classroom teaching and teaching awards, and so on. Regardless of who is defining it, however, without the pursuit of quality, it will be difficult to pursue a vision or improve a school or department. Quality depends on a variety of factors. Seymour (1992) addressed quality in higher education through various principles. For example:

- *Quality is continuous improvement.* "The challenge is to develop an organizational culture in which people accept the notion that change—or striving—must be considered constant" (p. 14).
- *Quality is leadership.* "The leadership must build strong consensus regarding quality and take every opportunity to reinforce that consensus" (p. 15). Quality is inclusive.
- *Quality is human resource development.* "It must become a part of the management function to help people learn their jobs and perform them better" (p. 16).
- *Quality is in the system.* "If improved quality is the goal, then the way to achieve it is to ask the people who work *in the system* to join with management to work *on the system*" (p. 17).

- *Quality is fear-reduction, recognition, and reward.* "The management of an organization should make a conscious investment in helping people perform their jobs better by reducing their fears and rewarding their quality-causing efforts" (p. 18).
- *Quality is teamwork.* "We have to organize ourselves into teams of people who work both in and on these [quality-improvement] processes" (p. 19). Again, quality includes various members of a community.
- *Quality is measurement.* "Continuous quality improvement requires a continuous flow of data [measurement]" (p. 19).
- *Quality is systematic problem-solving.* "People need to work together to generate objective data concerning processes in which they work and then apply that wisdom to a systematic methodology for improvement" (p. 20).

A school or department with a vision that includes quality and continuous improvement as benchmarks will increase its probability of effectiveness and success. Mediocrity is not the measure. High-quality performance is the key to any organization and the individuals who compose it.

Teamwork, shared identity, ongoing communication, recognition of others, delegation, and trust are all important to the promotion of quality in the academy. These principles must become part of the leader's mind, soul, and vision for success.

Summary

The crew of the *Endurance* survived their horrendous journey because they had a leader who, even under the most severe circumstances, recognized how important his leadership was to the survival of the crew. He did not run from his responsibility, but instead did everything in his power to maintain a vision of hope that manifested itself in a survival plan and, ultimately, rescue. Shakelton created a sense of purpose that led to teamwork, open communication, delegation, trust, caring, faith, and life itself. Although the most negative of situations within the academy fail to mirror the circumstances of Shakelton and his crew, the ideas and concepts that we have discussed within this chapter suggest how we can approach the future within our departments and schools. A good leader will have a balanced vision (such as those proposed by Boyer and the Kellogg Commission), will create and prioritize a set of principles, and will develop ways to operationalize the vision.

Administration of a school or department is tough work. As with Shakelton, it calls for passion, a sense of purpose, a bit of craziness, and, at times, an ability to respond to the unexpected. At the same time, it calls for a "game plan" and skilled leadership—skill in leading others to assess and improve their circumstances and the future of others. It calls for real community, where all members are devoted to promoting the welfare of society through their various emphases. It is a journey where the life-rafts don't have to be used—where we can feel secure about and be recognized for our contributions to our disciplines and to society.

About the Authors

Thomas J. Templin is head of the Department of Health, Kinesiology, and Leisure Studies at Purdue University. As a professor at the university since 1977, he has focused his research and writing on sport pedagogy and the socialization of physical educators. Most recently, he has focused on the administration of HKLS departments.

B. Don Franks is a professor in the Department of Kinesiology at the University of Maryland, where he has also served as chair. Previously, he has been coordinator of research laboratories at both the University of Illinois and Temple University, and a department chair at both the University of Tennessee and Louisiana State University.

References

Belasco, J. (1990). *Teaching the elephant to dance: Empowering change in your organization. New York: Crown.*

Boyer, E. (1990). *Scholarship reconsidered: Priorities of the professoriate. San Francisco: Jossey-Bass.*

Katzenbach, J., & Smith, D. (1993). The discipline of teams. *Harvard Business Review, 71*(2), 111-120.

Kellogg Commission on the Future of State and Land-Grant Universities. (1997). *Returning to our roots: The student experience.* Washington, DC: National Association of State Universities and Land-Grant Colleges.

Kellogg Commission on the Future of State and Land-Grant Universities. (1998a). *Returning to our roots: Student access.* Washington, DC: National Association of State Universities and Land-Grant Colleges.

Kellogg Commission on the Future of State and Land-Grant Universities. (1998b). *Returning to our roots: The engaged institution.* Washington, DC: National Association of State Universities and Land-Grant Colleges.

Kellogg Commission on the Future of State and Land-Grant Universities. (1999). *Returning to our roots: A learning society.* Washington, DC: National Association of State Universities and Land-Grant Colleges.

Kellogg Commission on the Future of State and Land-Grant Universities. (2000a). *Returning to our roots: Toward a coherent campus culture.* Washington, DC: National Association of State Universities and Land-Grant Colleges.

Kellogg Commission on the Future of State and Land-Grant Universities. (2000b). *Returning the covenant: Learning, discovery, and engagement in a new age and different world.* Washington, DC: National Association of State Universities and Land-Grant Colleges.

Kretchmar, R. (Ed.). (1999). The academy papers, no. 32: Telling our story [Special issue]. *Quest, 51*(2).

Moore, R. (1998). Building strong academic programs for the future: Practical experience at the University of Colorado–Boulder. *Quest, 50,* 198-205.

Nanus, B. (1992). *Visionary leadership: Creating a compelling sense of direction for your organization.* San Francisco: Jossey-Bass.

Peck, S. (1987). *The different drum: Community-making and peace.* New York: Touchstone.

Perkins, D. (2000). *Leading at the edge: Leadership lessons from the extraordinary saga of Shakelton's Antarctic expedition.* New York: American Management Association.

PEW Higher Education Round Table. (1996). Double agent. *Policy Perspectives, 6*(3), 1-12.

Reekie, S., & Wilkinson, S. (1997). Defensive no more! *The Chronicle of Physical Education in Higher Education, 8*(2), 1, 13.

Seymour, D. (1992). *On Q: Causing quality in higher education.* New York: Macmillan.

Templin, T. (2000). Departmental renewal: Reflections on the induction period of a new department head. *The Chronicle of Physical Education in Higher Education, 11*(2), 11-14.

Wilmore, J. (Ed.). (1998). The academy papers: Meeting the challenges of the 21st century in higher education [Special issue]. *Quest, 50*(2).

22 Knowing When Your Job Is Done and What to Do about It

Richard A. Swanson, *Professor, Department of Exercise and Sport Science, University of North Carolina at Greensboro*

Always be mindful that one's reputation for integrity will usually outlive one's accomplishments or mistakes.

⚬══ Richard A. Swanson

The decision to voluntarily leave a particular administrative position is a highly personal one that should not be taken lightly. For most people, it is a somewhat difficult decision because of the uncertainties involved. What is my motivation in leaving? Are other factors in my life playing a part in my decision? Have I completed what I set out to accomplish (or what I was charged with accomplishing) in my current position? Have I expended all of my political capital, such that I am no longer effective in this role? What will I do next? Will I be happy and fulfilled in another role? Do I want to continue in a different administrative capacity or return to the full-time professoriate? These and other questions float in and out of one's consciousness during the decision-making process, as well they should.

Rare is the department head or dean who has not, at one time or another, asked the question, "Is this what I really want to do for the remainder of my professional life?" This issue often raises its head when an especially knotty problem is looming or when the crush of too many deadlines competing for time and attention is creating high levels of stress. This may be particularly true in departments or schools that house programs in exercise science, physical education, health, dance, and recreation (even more so if intercollegiate athletics or intramural recreation is added to the mix). For instance, in addition to the normal personnel and curricular issues found in any academic unit, an administrator in these fields usually has sole or shared responsibility for a variety of facilities, some of which are used by several different programs. These facilities may include classrooms, laboratories, dance studios, gymnasiums, swimming pools, theaters, various outdoor facilities, and even clinical-service facilities for medical referrals, all with their attendant concerns for safety, box-office and billing procedures, and so forth. Mediating facility disputes between competing interests is often stressful for even the most skilled administrators. Add to that the constant concern for facility safety, fiscal responsibility, and other matters unique to these fields, and it is no wonder that such administrators often experience high levels of stress and burnout. Even without such stress, an administrator may still ask "Do I really want to continue in this role?" out of a simple desire for change. Regardless, serious reflection and analysis is required if one is to avoid regretting the jump to another role or staying on while ignoring signs of increasing dissatisfaction or boredom that may lead to an eventual deterioration in performance. For obvious reasons, it is always preferable to make such a decision during a non-crisis period.

Administrators make the decision to vacate a position for a variety of reasons. The following are some of the most common: (1) when the passion for the job is gone; (2) when the mission or goals set before one at the beginning of an appointment have been accomplished; (3) when health concerns for oneself or one's family seem to dictate the need for a less stressful role; (4) when other family needs or crises demand a higher priority than the job will allow; (5) when philosophical, professional, or personal differences with one's administrative superior(s) or the faculty become irresolvable; (6) when other professional opportunities for administrative advancement become available; (7) when the desire to return to full-time professorial status becomes greater than the desire to remain in administration; and (8) when one determines that the time for professional retirement has arrived. While some of the above might be viewed as positive reasons for ending an administrative tenure (fulfillment of goals, administrative promotion, returning to the joy of teaching and research, retirement) and others as negative (loss of passion, illness, conflict), the fact is that all can result in positive outcomes for both administrators and those with whom they work.

Loss of Passion

Losing one's enthusiasm for a particular role is not an uncommon occurrence. Certainly, not everyone experiences such loss. Most of us know individuals who have carried on in the same department-head or dean position for many years with no apparent loss of excitement. Their energy levels remain consistently high, new ideas and ways of doing things sprout forth each year like new leaves on trees, and their leadership remains strong. For many of us, however, a long tenure in the same administrative position eventually takes its toll. For some, this period is only four or five years, while others are content for a decade or more after their original appointment. Certainly, the level of stress experienced can affect the joy one feels in a job. Year after year of seemingly intractable problems can take their toll on anyone. The steady diet of deadlines, personnel issues, facility conflicts, budget constraints, working on other persons' agendas, and so forth can make one long for the relative freedom of faculty, who appear to have more control over teaching goals, research topics, and even many service commitments. Let's face it, administration as a lifelong career is not for everyone! For others, however, the burnout may be job-specific, and a change to another administrative position may lead to continued success.

Whatever the cause, the loss of passion for a particular role has serious consequences for the administrator, the unit's faculty, and the institution as a whole. The administrator grows increasingly frustrated, despondent, and ineffective in the job. The faculty suffer from a lack of administrative attention and departmental stagnation. The institution as a whole suffers when any single unit begins to fall into disarray. For this reason, it is the obligation of the administrator in question to acknowledge the problem, engage in serious reflection and analysis, and either commit to attempting a renewal of enthusiasm or gracefully move on to the next stage of professional life. The well-being of the individual, the unit, and the institution depend on it.

It may well be that enthusiasm and passion for the job is waning because the major tasks of the position have been completed. New administrators should have a reasonable idea of what sorts of things are expected of them. What needs immediate attention: rebuilding the faculty, establishing new programs, managing enrollment, mediating in "turf" controversies between faculty, programs, or departments? What are the more long-range goals: providing leadership in long-range planning, assessing possible construction or renovation of facilities, reorganizing the unit? If after several years all of these goals appear to have been completed, it is time for major assessment. Here is where excellent lines of communication between the administrator and her or his supervisor come in handy. If annual performance reviews have been carried out and annual reports carefully constructed, a serious conversation between the two persons should reveal if the immediate charge has been met. At the same time, it is important to determine if there are additional goals to be set and if the person's skills match up with what has to be done. No matter how successful a particular administrator may have been in accomplishing the original goals, it may well be that someone with a different administrative personality and set of skills is needed to move the department to the next level or through the next stage of its life.

Mission Accomplished

Thus it may be time to consider making a change if:

- the initial tasks are truly finished *and*
- no new, attractive challenges appear to be on the horizon *and*
- the person is unexcited about presiding over a unit that may require only caretaking, *or*
- the position now appears to require different talents.

Conflict

While disagreements between administrators and their faculty or their superiors are not uncommon, such conflict occasionally becomes so serious and protracted that the administrator is rendered ineffective. Generally, conflict this severe is the result of a buildup of distrust or dislike over a long period of time. Rarely is it the result of a single event, unless that action was so egregious that trust or confidence in the person's abilities or integrity is destroyed (e.g., an administrator deliberately lying to the faculty about a situation or falsifying a report to the chief academic officer of the institution). While such actions sometimes result in immediate removal from office, in many cases even such outrageous behavior is simply noted and then filed away, both formally and informally, for use in judging future behavior.

More commonly, distrust is built up over time by a series of actions or misunderstandings, or by differences in personality, administrative style, and perceptions of the goals and mission of the unit or institution. Whatever the reason, if it appears that the relationship is beyond repair, then it is probably the appropriate time to prepare for leaving the post.

The Grass Really May Be Greener

If any of the above conditions applies, it may not necessarily dictate the end of one's administrative career. Assuming that one's desire to continue in a managerial role remains strong, a change in location and type of position may be warranted. If this is the case, the individual has the advantage of experience to look at subsequent opportunities in a more sophisticated way and to make the next move a successful one. Ideally, the person now has a better understanding of his or her own strengths and shortcomings. A look at past successes as well as those situations that might have been handled differently is absolutely essential if one is to improve the likelihood of success in a future position. Conversations with trusted faculty and other administrators are useful in this endeavor. "Trusted" does not necessarily exclude those who might have been opposed to your policies or style or who might be supportive of your decision to leave. The important consideration is whether or not their truthfulness, judgment, and sense of fairness can be trusted. The fact that a person disagrees with you does not necessarily make them an enemy.

Experience should also dictate those things to look for in a new position that will best ensure a good fit between administrator and institution. A desperate desire to vacate a current position can sometimes cloud one's judgment concerning a new one. Thus honest dialogue in the interview process is absolutely necessary, whether it be with faculty, administrative staff, the president, or the chancellor. Do you agree with the institution's academic philosophy, values, and the way it treats its employees and constituents? Is the faculty of the unit largely united or hopelessly divided regarding goals and vision? Is the central administration visibly and sincerely supportive of the unit, its mission, and its faculty? Is this truly a place where you want to invest an important portion of your life over the next several years?

Return to the Faculty

The motivation for leaving administration and returning to the faculty may be prompted by a number of factors. Hopefully, it is because the individual loves the teaching, research, and scholarly activities that are difficult to carry on while serving as an administrator. At the risk of oversimplification and stereotyping, it has been this writer's experience that administrators in the disciplines encompassed within what is traditionally called "health, physical education, recreation, and dance" (HPERD) have far more administrative responsibilities than those in many of the liberal arts (e.g., accreditation requirements; career opportunities for students; facility management; changes in the nature of the profession; constant reorganization of curricula in the various programs to better meet professional and societal needs). Thus HPERD administrators' desire to resume more traditional academic careers as members of the full-time professoriate can become overwhelming. They miss the joy of the classroom experience or of conducting research. They long to set their own agenda each day rather than having it determined primarily by the needs of others. They may have thoroughly enjoyed their time as administrators but found that their enthusiasm has begun to waver.

Fortunately, an administrator who also holds rank as a tenured faculty member has the luxury of making such a change in career direction. Within the world of business, it is rarely possible for a person to reverse directions on the corporate ladder in this manner. The rungs below are usually filled with younger climbers, and one who remains on one step for too long becomes a clog in the machine and must either continue to climb or be forced to leave the company. An academic administrator, however, can usually decide to return to her or his academic roots and, presumably, pick up the pieces and carry on.

Not every administrator who returns to the faculty does so because of burnout or a yearning to teach and write again. For some, the decision is more or less forced, either due to the institution's desire for a change in leadership or to a personal health or family crisis. While the decision to leave may not be a totally free one in such cases, there are choices to make regarding how one accepts this decision and deals with its consequences.

As in the case of administrative burnout, persons who have contracted health problems serious enough to affect their job performance must strongly consider removing themselves from the position for their own good as well as for that of the unit. A brief leave of absence might well suffice for many minor as well as some major health problems (e.g., heart attack, stroke, surgery, radiation and chemotherapy treatments). If there are serious residual effects that result in periodic relapses or a permanent loss of energy, however, the stress and demands of academic administration may well prove to be too much for even the most strong-willed individual. To attempt to carry on in such a case will surely detract from the performance of one's duties and may prove detrimental to one's health.

A prolonged family crisis (e.g., physical or mental illness, marital difficulties, caring for an aged parent) can exact the same toll. Each case is unique, of course, and individuals handle such stresses and medical problems differently. Thus the above examples are not hard and fast rules that determine when a person *must* leave an administrative role. Recovery rates from serious illnesses and coping abilities during other crises are very individualized. When such situations arise, however, a constant self-monitoring process should be carried out. In addition, it is important to let one's administrative superiors and/or a trusted colleague know about these situations in order to garner moral and emotional support and, perhaps, assistance in the monitoring process. These individuals can be helpful in determining if and when the department or the administrator is beginning to suffer from the strain. In cases of physical illness, this knowledge will usually be fairly public within the unit. Yet one's emotional health may not be readily apparent to others—especially faculty and staff—until one's behavior is affected. Hopefully, the individual will be aware of the problem before this occurs and will have sought professional or other appropriate assistance. The point is, administrators have an obligation to others as well as to themselves, and they need to be prepared for the possibility of such situations long before they occur—after all, this *is* a high-stress occupation.

In the case of dismissal from a position by administrative fiat, you must decide how to accept this action and the subsequent forced return to the faculty that you may have been leading. While you may not have been the one to make the decision to leave your post, you are the only one who can control how you proceed from this point. There may well be feelings of embarrassment, pain, anger, and bitterness. These feelings are real and cannot be ignored. They must be acknowledged and dealt with, possibly with professional counseling, so that they do not get in the way of effective teaching and relationships with your colleagues in the department. The welfare of the students and your own mental health are at stake.

It should be noted that negative emotions may be present whether one leaves an administrative post due to illness or due to dismissal; in both cases, the person may feel forced out of the position. More often than not, however, an administrator with medical problems can count on support and empathy from fellow faculty members. This might also be true in the case of dismissal if the faculty had positive relations with the administrator and the firing was perceived as unfair (e.g., at the hands of a distrusted higher administrator). Such collegial support can certainly ease one's return to the faculty, even if the person wishes to remain in administration and plans to seek such positions elsewhere in the near future. A fired administrator who feels little or no support from the faculty may well be faced with the decision to seek a new position at another institution rather quickly. Whatever the case, a commitment to one's students and to the work of the department is essential. A decision to honor that commitment is imperative if the former administrator is to rebuild his or her own self-confidence, gain any support from colleagues, and regain a sense of purpose and personal happiness.

CASE STUDY: One Person's Decision to Leave Administration

As one who made the decision several years ago to leave administration and return to the full-time faculty at the same institution, this writer can attest to both the simplicity and the complexity of the move. After two decades as a department head, assistant director, and dean at three universities, I was emotionally and intellectually ready to leave my final position as dean of a highly respected school of health and human performance. Yet I wrestled with the final decision over the course of a year before finally announcing my intention to step down three years hence. The announcement was made at the time of a regularly scheduled five-year review. There was work to be done in getting the unit settled into a new building, and it seemed appropriate to complete that transition before forcing everyone to work through a change in leadership. In hindsight, however, three years as an announced lame duck was at least one year too long, and I would now recommend no more than one or two.

I'm not certain of the exact moment when I became aware of my desire to leave the administrative fold and return to full-time faculty status. It was a gradual awareness stimulated by specific events. For instance, a four-day period working on a research project at another campus left me feeling refreshed and intellectually stimulated. I recall feeling puzzled by this awareness because my administrative life at the time was challenging and stimulating as well. We were in the midst of planning the new HPERD facility. While fraught with its own set of problems and frustrations, such a project was, nevertheless, the kind of opportunity that most academic administrators dream will come their way at least once in their career. I was enormously fulfilled in a professional sense. Still, on the drive home I determined that some day I would want to return to full-time teaching and research.

Over the next several years, this desire was an occasional but insistent thought. Not surprisingly, the notion sometimes came when I was working through particularly difficult personnel or budget problems, or when I was juggling so many balls simultaneously that the fear of disaster became almost overwhelming. Undoubtedly, these are normal feelings in times of heavy stress. Some people thrive on this kind of challenge throughout their career. For me, the exhilaration derived from contributions made through administrative service gradually began to fade, and I yearned for the more individually focused life of teacher-scholar. As the date for moving into our new and renovated facilities drew near (along with the approach of my tenth year as dean), it seemed appropriate to begin giving serious consideration to leaving the post. Other important tasks had also been successfully completed (e.g., reorganization of the school and the building of a new faculty following a period of numerous retirements). Feeling a sense of accomplishment along with the aforementioned fatigue, I shared my intentions with the faculty, the provost, and the chancellor.

My decision brought with it many of the same anxieties discussed earlier in this chapter. How long will it take to get up to speed in my field of study? Is it even possible to get back in touch with that field after many years away from the daily discipline of reading, research, and dialogue with colleagues around the country? How useful can I be to the department as a faculty member? How will my new faculty colleagues receive me after knowing me only in the role of dean? Will I really enjoy my new role as much as I have savored the anticipation?

A period of eight years has now passed since my exit as dean. I can happily confirm that my colleagues have been wonderfully kind, welcoming, and helpful. This has been especially true in regard to my learning to work within the policies, procedures, forms, and customs of the department and the school, some of which I had helped to create as dean (perhaps every administrator should occasionally be forced to deal with his or her own directives from the position of the consumer). My level of energy and enthusiasm has remained high, and I am thoroughly enjoying my work.

What, then, have I learned since assuming my new role? What adjustments have been required? There are, first of all, the obvious external rewards that one no longer receives. In most cases, there may be a dramatic salary adjustment as one moves from a 12-month to a 9-month appointment, with perhaps the accompanying loss of any administrative stipend. This is an adjustment that requires advance planning, just as one would plan for any major life change such as retirement, marriage, or children.

The loss of a private secretarial staff that always put the dean's work first has been a major adjustment for more than one former administrator. Suddenly you find yourself part of a group of faculty sharing a secretary, opening your own mail, and typing much of your own work (if you don't wish to wait in line).

The move to a smaller, perhaps less elegant office has been an unexpected shock to many who thought that their physical surroundings would be of little importance to them. Considering my own personality and recognizing that I work most effectively in a neat, pleasant office environment, I tried to plan ahead. Using university resources and personal funds, I created a smaller, but warm and inviting, office that is comfortable for the way in which I prefer to work, minus the stress of the dean's office. As dean, I had a *large*, beautiful office. As a professor, I have a *small*, beautiful office. At this stage of life, I prefer small.

A real positive in all of this has been the tremendous reduction in the amount of daily mail; my "to read" file is no longer filled with reports from various on- and off-campus offices. On the other hand, as I had been forewarned, there is a sudden realization that you are out of the information loop. If information is power, then it becomes very clear that the power has shifted.

A common concern, of course, is that a former dean or department head who remains on the faculty will be a thorn in the side of the new administrator or simply despondent at the sight of another person occupying the office and possibly redirecting the focus of the school or reversing existing policies. Thus it is important to make it clear that while you wish to be helpful to the new administrator, you will not be offering unsolicited advice. Rather, you will be available for consultation on any issues that the new administrator wishes to discuss. As for despondency over changes, I can only wish for others to be as fortunate as I have been. Our new dean is full of energy, intelligence, common sense, good humor, character, and grace. My adjustment was, therefore, easy and comfortable. The school is in good hands and moving forward on new challenges. A former dean can ask no more than that.

This is just one person's story. My own decision is not correct for everyone, just as my experience will not necessarily be that of others. If anything is to be learned here, it is:

- first, to trust your own instincts;

- second, to talk with others who have taken a similar path (while you are still in the decision-making stage); and

- third, to carefully think through and plan each step of the transition process, from arranging personal finances, to creating a new office environment, to developing at least a two-year teaching and scholarship agenda that is energizing and motivating.

There is always the danger of experiencing a vacuum as you move from an environment of daily deadlines and unexpected crises to one in which you have more control over your agenda, yet are required to exhibit more self-discipline. In other words, you should plan a realistic but full schedule.

This section has been adapted from R. A. Swanson (1993), "When to Say When: On One Dean's Decision to Return to the Professoriate," *The Chronicle of Physical Education in Higher Education*, 4(3), 4, 15.

When to say when? Only the individual and his or her circumstances can determine that. Eventually, though, it comes for almost everyone, one way or another. Of utmost importance is remembering that the administrative position is a public trust. The welfare of the department, school, or college is paramount. This is not to make light of the welfare of the individual in question. Most of the time, however, what is best for one is also best for the other. Most department heads and deans are not happy if they remain past their time. Therefore, constant monitoring of one's own feelings and instincts, thorough periodic reviews of the unit and its leadership, and dialogue with trusted colleagues and friends are essential elements in this aspect of career decision-making. Perhaps the best administrative decision of all is knowing when to say when.

Summary

Richard A. Swanson, professor in the Department of Exercise and Sport Science at the University of North Carolina at Greensboro, was a successful department head and dean for 24 of his 36 years in higher education.

About the Author

23 Preparing to Be an Administrator

Steve Estes, *Associate Professor and Chair, Department of Exercise and Sport Science, East Carolina University*

When in doubt, consult! When consulting, trust yourself!

⚬══✦══⚬ Steve Estes

Two of the most challenging roles in higher education are those of chair and dean. Both types of administrators must deal with the expectations and desires of every university constituency: students, faculty, administrators, alumni, and staff. In order to succeed in their leadership roles, both must perform many of the same tasks (e.g., teaching, research, service). Yet the two roles are also substantially different. For instance, the role of the chair has been described as "paradoxical": a leader, yet led, an administrator who is administered, a first among equals who exists at the pleasure of both one's supervisors and one's peers (Tucker, 1992). The duties of chairs include department governance, instruction, faculty affairs, student affairs, external and internal communications, budgeting, office management, and professional development. Yet chairs do not have the explicit authority to dictate action in any of these roles. Chairs can be seen as the sergeants of the university, responsible for implementing what these institutions say they are all about.

In contrast, deans often contend that chairing a department is more difficult than serving as dean of a school or college, though they note that this difference is more in the pace of administering than in the level of task difficulty. Deans are responsible for implementing the mission of the institution, and they must "use" departments to get the job done. Doing so requires significant delegation and leadership skills and a well-developed sense of mission. When describing the qualities of a good dean, chairs often reply that they do not know what the dean does—until there is a problem, and the dean is there to help! How does a potential dean acquire these skills? It would appear that chairing a department would provide some training, but serving as a dean is also a leap into uncharted territory, where decisions to nourish or starve units require the use of criteria that chairs do not have at their disposal.

Two questions should be asked if the above comments regarding chairs and deans are in any way true. The first is: why would anyone want one of these positions? The second is: assuming any rational person *would* want one of these positions, how on earth could one possibly prepare for them?! Faculty take on administrative positions for many reasons, among them the desire to be good at the job of leading their peers in health, kinesiology, and leisure-studies (HKLS) units. Hopefully, candidates see administrative positions as creative ones, where the chair or dean has the authority to facilitate the development of opportunities and programs for students and faculty. In this respect, administration in HKLS units is similar to administration in other academic units. Yet the scope of duties for HKLS administrators is larger than that for administrators in the traditional academic disciplines. HKLS units provide academic as well as professional opportunities for students. HKLS units also integrate the humanities, social sciences, and sciences, whereas more traditional academic units tend to emphasize one of these three. Finally, HKLS units often offer significant services (e.g., student recreation, general education courses, faculty fitness programs) that are surprisingly large in scope. HKLS administrators, in effect, can be seen as "mini-provosts," only without large budgets.

Where do chairs and deans come from? Almost all begin as faculty members, but the similarities end there. With respect to chairing, some faculty secure the position in national searches (21 percent), but most (79 percent) come from within their department (Mawson, 1998). Other times, it becomes a given faculty member's "turn" to serve as chair when no other faculty can or will perform these duties (1.9 percent of all new chairs). Deans are more often selected in national searches, and almost all deans have performed the duties of a chair in one of the departments housed in their school or college.

Whatever your reason for pursuing a chair or dean position, and whatever your background, you will find that there are a number of positive steps you can take to prepare yourself for securing an administrative position. In doing so, you will increase the possibility that you will be hired, whether you are an internal or external candidate. Part anecdote, part personal experience, and part research, this chapter will provide you with a practical guide for preparing to serve as a chair or dean.

Growing into an Administrative Position

Understand universities and their missions. The first step in preparing for an administrative position is to understand what such a position is. In my experience, and in conversations with deans about their experiences, I have found that chairs and deans make the administrative decisions that help university missions "come to life." If this is the case, then your first step is to study your university's mission, or the mission of the university where you will be applying, in order to help you understand exactly what it is you will be managing. It will help if you study university missions in general. You may be surprised at what you find in such an exercise[1]. To state the obvious, universities vary greatly in mission. Liberal-arts institutions are very different animals from research institutions, community colleges, and comprehensive institutions. One of your most important roles will be to articulate and justify the mission of your unit to your faculty, to the school/college that houses it, and to the university as a whole.

You will find that your experiences as a faculty member will guide you in expressing the mission of your unit to the outside world. Mobley (1999) noted that this is one of the strengths of prospective administrators; they usually have a good academic record, "a very solid understanding of the university [and] the customs of the academic community, and a faculty perspective on issues" (p. 1) Another of your key roles will be to guide your faculty in ways that fulfill the university mission and the plans of your chief academic officer or dean. In any case, you will not be able to do your job if you do not know what your university's mission is or how your unit fits into that mission.

This broad philosophical understanding will manifest itself in specific, day-to-day operations. For instance, some faculty will wish to teach, some to research, and still others to focus on serving the university and community. It will be your job to both guide and facilitate these wishes, and to do so in the context of the university's mission. Yet, you will not be able to fulfill this role unless you know where your particular university is going, and why. Furthermore, in order to obtain scarce resources, you will find that it is very helpful to be able to compare your unit to others at your university and to similar units at other universities. You should also understand and be able to articulate the history of your unit and institution and the teaching, service, and research styles that support your mission. Some excellent resources for learning about university missions are Boyer's (1990) *Scholarship Reconsidered: Priorities of the Professoriate* and Glassick, Huber, and Maeroff's (1997) *Scholarship Assessed: Evaluation of the Professoriate.* These books summarize succinctly what universities are about and describe faculty roles, university missions, and their relationship to teaching, research, and service. Scholars in many disciplines, including HKLS, have discussed and interpreted these works at length[2].

Study how you manage. A second step in preparing to be an administrator is to try to understand how you operate on the job. Potential deans will usually have their past experiences as chairs on which to reflect, while potential chairs will have fewer management experiences to study. I have found that the chair's position is primarily a managerial one, and that it is a far more important management position than most realize. Indeed, it is the management position that is most central to operationalizing a university's mission; studies show that chairs make as many as *80 percent* of all administrative decisions in higher education (Knight & Holen, 1985).

Both positions are, ultimately, management positions; thus, examining your own management style is a valuable practice. There are many excellent management books on the market (Furnham, 1992; Keirsey & Bates, 1998). Pick one that provides psychological questionnaires that can help you understand your management style (e.g., the Myers-Briggs system)[3]. This exercise will reveal that you have some strengths—and some weaknesses. More importantly, though, you will see that you will be good at some of the tasks of a chair, and will need to work at others. For instance, I've had good experiences in leading groups, building teams, and working on mission and vision. In contrast, budgeting, student files, and paperwork associated with personnel are areas where I need help. I find it best to have staff do the latter tasks while I concentrate on the former, but all of the work just described is important (just ask any administrator who has ever neglected to process a necessary faculty travel reimbursement!).

Managerial positions are multifaceted, and call for many different skills. It is no surprise, then, that so many chief executive officers in corporations come from broad liberal-arts backgrounds (Neff & Ogden, 1998). The ability to express yourself both orally and in writing, to use mathematics to express various budget relationships, to understand the relationships of groups to the whole, and so forth, are essential tools for any chair, regardless of one's field. Neff and Ogden's description of the ideal CEO is equally applicable to the university administrator, who "must be a quick thinker and eloquent speaker, capable of calming concerned [faculty, students, staff, and deans]; satisfying government agencies; inspiring confidence among the analyst community; making friends with the press; and skillfully working with competitors interested in forming strategic alliances" (p. 32). Thus, you must prepare yourself, as best you can, to see many perspectives that you have not seen before and to articulate these perspectives to everyone who comes in contact with your unit.

Be a good faculty member. A good record of teaching, research, and service is expected of any potential administrator. If you are to be "first among your peers," then you would be well advised to have demonstrated competence in these areas before seeking such a position. While it is not necessary to be the very best at a given institution in any one of these areas, it is very helpful if you are an accomplished teacher, scholar, and service-provider during your tenure as a faculty member. The credibility gained among your faculty as being "one of us" will prove most helpful.

More specifically, this often means having been promoted to professor prior to becoming an administrator. While there are many associate professors who chair departments (but few who are deans), most administrators find it difficult to focus on the teaching, research, and service activities necessary for promotion. Don't plan on leaving the faculty entirely once you occupy an administrative position, though. Chairs and deans usually advise that once you are in an administrative position, you should maintain some level of research, teaching, and service in order to stay "grounded" in the field (Mobley, 1999). In so doing, you will know firsthand the problems that your faculty face in their everyday work and, again, enhance your credibility.

Study chairing and "deaning." While there are no surefire steps that one can take to become an administrator, there is a body of knowledge that one can study in order to prepare for and obtain such a position. The reference list at the end of this chapter is a good place to begin. My favorite resources for chairing include Dustin's (1993) *For the Good of the Order: Administering Academic Programs in Higher Education,* a series of essays written by recreation and leisure-studies chairs on their administrative experiences; Seagren, Creswell, and Wheeler's (1993) *The Department Chair: New Roles, Responsibilities, and Challenges,* a report that summarizes scholarly studies of chairing; Tucker's (1992) *Chairing the Academic Department: Leadership Among Peers,* the most in-depth study of chairing that I've read; and a series of articles in *The Chronicle of Physical Education in Higher Education* by Mawson (1998), Mobley (1999), and Dunn (1999) that discuss selecting, developing, and evaluating department chairs. Two excellent books on deans include Morris' (1981) *Deaning: Middle Management in Academe* and Rosovsky's (1990) *The University: An Owner's Manual.* All of these works will

Specific Steps in Preparing for an Administrative Position

provide you with helpful information in preparing for, and succeeding in, administrative positions.

Get practical administrative experience. Potential deans have prior administrative experiences, and can describe those experiences in their vitae and during interviews. Potential chairs, though, often lack administrative experience. Once I decided that I wanted to apply for chair positions, one of my first tasks was to look for management opportunities at the college where I taught. There is no substitute for administrative experience, and I had little of it. Usually, however, such experience can be gained without too much searching. Every university at which I have worked has been "under-administered," meaning that there is likely an administrator on your campus who can use a hand. My experience as director of a center for instructional technology, as faculty senate chair, and as a discipline coordinator all helped me understand many of the decisions that chairs face. Most often, these decisions fall into one of three general areas: curriculum, personnel, or budget. The literature supports this observation. Mobley (1999), for instance, argued that the administrative areas that potential chairs need to work on the most are personnel management, budgeting, and development/fundraising. If you can gain some significant level of administrative experience in these areas, then your application will be enhanced. And don't limit your administrative experience to your university; chairing committees or presiding over your professional society at the state, regional, or national level also provide excellent administrative experiences and networking opportunities.

Learn the curriculum process. Curricular decisions are generally considered to be the purview of the faculty. Chairs and deans, however, sign off on new curricula and other curricular changes, encourage faculty to develop courses and degree programs, facilitate and oversee the curriculum-development process, and promote certain curricula over others (by the manner in which they assign staff and resources). To the extent that you may have worked with curriculum in this manner, your ability to move into the chair position is improved. You should join (or, preferably, chair) department, school, or university curriculum committees to learn the process of editing and approving curricula. Getting faculty together to read proposals, to move these proposals through committee (especially when there are significant disagreements), and to guide these proposals through the many institutional reviews is good practice for the type of leadership that chairs must exhibit. If you can acquire the management skills that curriculum-committee chairs possess, then you will be well on your way to understanding the nature of the skills (persuasion, argument, rhetoric, wheedling, cajoling!) that administrators often use.

Understand the personnel process. The people that departments hire, grant tenure to, and schedule will make or break you as an administrator. Personnel decisions are made with both faculty and administrative input, and chairs, followed by deans, initiate the administrative process. Chairs and deans do not grant tenure, promote, and award merit pay, but their concurrence or non-concurrence with the various decisions of personnel committees (PCs) are highly regarded and almost always serve as the implicit "final word" on such matters. To prepare for these decisions, it is helpful to work on your department's PC and, if possible, chair it. Working with your chair or dean on these decisions will provide you with valuable observations as to how this process works at your institution and at all institutions in general. Indeed, a good PC chair is worth his or her weight in gold; he or she provides advice to the department chair on who is productive and who is not, reminds the chair of important due dates, edits the language used in tenure letters, and sits with the chair when untenured faculty are advised of their progress. There are other experiences that one can seek out to learn about making personnel decisions, but the best experiences are found on a PC. Similarly, working with your dean on personnel issues provides insight into how higher-level administrators prioritize and allocate positions.

Learn how to budget. Chairs and deans reward some programs and strangle others, and an important tool in this process is the allocation of financial resources. Budgeting is not difficult, but it can be tedious, and there is no substitute for experience. Academic administrators are usually provided fewer budgetary resources than they would like, and the allocation of scarce resources has been known to drive otherwise productive administrators out of the job. Chairs and deans are now being asked to generate resources, and professional meetings usually include sessions on how to work with external grant agencies and procure contracts that increase discretionary monies. If you have the ability to generate lots of money, then your budgeting duties will be a lot easier. In fact, it is amazing just how highly regarded your administrative skills will become if you can generate enough money to provide for the professional travel of all of your faculty!

The types of experiences that help one learn about budgeting are available in all colleges and universities. Running a small center (e.g., a center for faculty professional development or international studies) is a good start. Serving as treasurer in your professional societies or on faculty senates can provide you with an understanding of how universities allocate funds. A word about keeping track of university funds: oftentimes, university accounting becomes quite Byzantine. University-designed computing systems make accounts difficult to read, and sometimes it is hard to know how much money one actually has. Too often, one's budget arrives well into the academic year, which can delay much-needed purchases and make the hiring of graduate assistants and part-time faculty an exercise in crisis management. Accounting systems that post the same purchase five times in various approval stages are not unusual. Administrative staff across campus can be lifesavers as they aid you in tracking your funds, so learn how to work with them and cultivate the friendship of those who make budget decisions on your campus. Walking your own grants through the accounting system is one of the best methods of learning how to generate and spend money. Pay attention to the process, and get to know the people who make it happen.

Get mentors. Prior to acquiring a new administrative position, you should look for mentors, both in professional societies and in administrative positions at your institution. Often, your chair and dean will need help in their duties, so ask them if there are any tasks that you could fulfill. They will be grateful for the help and, like other professionals, willing to tell you about their job. If your unit head cannot or will not help you in this area, look for other administrators at your university who would like to work with you. It has been my experience that there is *always* at least one such administrator, and the more senior, the better. Two mentors are better than one; you will find that there are campus networks that facilitate administrative work, so tap into them. Early and regular breakfast or lunch "bull sessions" are the best; the anecdotes of your mentors will shape you in ways that are invaluable in both the application process and on the job. Remember that professionals in organizational development use mentoring because they know that it works so well.

If you secure a new position at a different university, find a mentor there. The advice of a former administrative colleague is invaluable, if for no other reason than getting a sense of institutional history. You will not believe how helpful this information is until you have to make a decision that requires a good sense of the peculiarities of your new unit.

Mentors also come in the form of peers. Be aware that the social aspects of administrative positions are exceptionally important. The work of the chair or dean is greatly facilitated by the ability to communicate with administrators in similar positions. As a unit head, you will come to value the support of colleagues experiencing similar problems on the job, if for no other reason than it helps in those lonely moments that any leader experiences. Organizations such as the College and University Administrators Council (CUAC) provide the support and socialization that can help make your administrative position an enjoyable one.

Once you have obtained an administrative position, you should work to develop an internal support group within your unit. The type of help you can get on personnel, budget, and curriculum issues (and on institutional history) are invaluable. If there are active faculty at your institution who have served as administrators for your unit in the past, seek them out and make them part of your executive team. You will find that weekly breakfast meetings with no agenda other than to talk about work may be the only opportunity you have to do the "mission/vision thing" that you had hoped would occupy all of your time as an administrator.

Join professional administrative societies. Establish a professional network; professional societies such as the National Association for Physical Education in Higher Education (NAPEHE), CUAC, and the American Association for Higher Education (AAHE) are good places to start. While a personal mentor will help you with the specifics of administration at your institution, a professional society provides you with more general ideas that can be applied to any institution. You will find that there is no substitute for working with other HKLS administrators; they have experienced problems similar to those that you will face in the future. The psychological support that is provided through such interactions is exceptionally valuable. These associations can also help you obtain future administrative positions.

Know your boss's job. One of the best pieces of advice given to me regarding chairing was, "It is your job to make your dean look good." This truism applies to deans as well. Understanding the job of your immediate administrative superior will help you obtain such a position down the road[4]. In its most superficial reading, this comment reduces administration to doing whatever it takes to make your boss happy. But a richer reading implies a thorough understanding of the mission of your college or school as seen through the eyes of your boss, and it can help prepare you for that higher position, should you aspire to it. At the very least, you will be able to describe in your job interview how you will facilitate your immediate superior's goals, which most often are the same as your own.

Apply, apply, apply. Begin applying for positions. It may take several years before the correct position comes along for you. You will find that the qualities of a specific administrative position will vary according to the needs of the given unit and institution. You will have skills that fit some institutions and faculties (and deans and provosts!) better than others. Don't be discouraged when you find that your "dream" department, school, or college doesn't select you—it may be a gift in disguise. There are excellent units that do not have the reputation of those in high-profile research institutions. These outstanding units may effectively fulfill their mission without many of the problems that more famous institutions have. Use all of the available resources to find out which units and institutions are searching for chairs and deans. *The Chronicle of Higher Education* remains one of the best resources; recently, however, web and e-mail databases such as *Opportunities in Physical Education and Related Areas (OPERA)* (www.napehe.org), its *Physical Education E-mail Directory* (found at the same web address), and the job database maintained by Human Kinetics (www.hkusa.com) have been developed that are free, current, and accurate.

Study leadership. The principles of leadership apply to academic administrative positions as much as they do to businesses. Yet one of the surprising characteristics of the academy is that its administrators rarely have true authority, at least of the type that academics associate with their business peers. So managing in academia is done more through collaborative leadership than through command. For instance, I have found that even when I have the authority to make a unilateral decision (e.g., while scheduling faculty teaching assignments), I am reluctant to impose my decision without significant consultation; I immediately sense that the consequences of this "imposition" would cause more problems than it would solve. Like other chairs, I find that I spend much of my time convincing those who report to me, and those to whom I report, of the merits of my ideas. You will find that your authority as an academic administrator is based more on your character and knowledge than on the statutory basis of your position. As Mobley (1999) and many others have reminded us, there is a difference between doing things right (managing) and doing the right things (leading). Chairs and deans do both, and a careful study of leadership will help you understand the difference.

| Summary | The above discussion is merely one more in a growing list that can prepare faculty for two of the most challenging administrative positions, excluding the role of the president, within the university. My advice—some of it personal, some anecdotal, and some scholarly—can help you begin this preparatory process. But I would like to conclude on a motivational note: these jobs are worth the effort! No matter how long you occupy one of these positions, you will never be the same after you obtain one. You will grow in ways you never thought possible, and you will probably be the better for it. Good luck! |

1   While you may be surprised at what you find, it is more likely that, as a potential administrator, you have always been interested in university missions. For instance, Mobley (1999) argued that new chairs characteristically bring a "good understanding of the university" to the chair position. I don't think that this characteristic is a coincidence.

2   For a discussion of Boyer's work in kinesiology, see the special issue of *Quest* (1996, volume 48, number 2) devoted to his *Scholarship Reconsidered*. Boyer's keynote address to the National Association for Physical Education in Higher Education is included in this issue; among other things, it summarizes the themes of Glassick et al.'s (1997) *Scholarship Assessed*. Other articles in this special issue discuss the missions of various kinds of universities (liberal arts, comprehensive, doctoral, and research) and other aspects of scholarship in kinesiology. The fields of health and leisure studies have been similarly influenced by these works of Boyer and Glassick et al.

3   Many such questionnaires are now available on the web. Using the words "MeyersBriggs" in a web search, I found the *Keirsey Temperament Sorter II*, an on-line questionnaire that assigns the test-taker to one of the Meyers-Briggs personality types, accompanied by easily understood analyses of the results.

4   My favorite book on this subject is Rosovsky's (1990) *The University: An Owner's Manual*. Rosovsky was dean of the Faculty of Arts and Sciences at Harvard University, and he chaired the university's Department of Economics before that. His insights into how universities work, the problems and successes he encountered, and the experience of serving as a dean will all be helpful to those who want to understand this role. Another good resource is Morris' (1981) *Deaning: Middle management in academe*. This book is especially interesting in that many of the jobs described by Morris in 1981 as the dean's responsibility are now within the purview of the chair.

Notes

Steve Estes is an associate professor in, and chair of, the Department of Exercise and Sport Science at East Carolina University. He has been involved in higher education administration for over three years.

About the Author

Boyer, E. (1990). *Scholarship reconsidered: Priorities of the professoriate*. Princeton, NJ: The Carnegie Foundation for the Advancement of Teaching.

Dunn, J. (1999). Evaluating the department chair. *The Chronicle of Physical Education in Higher Education,10*(2), 1, 12-14.

Dustin, D. (1993). *For the good of the order: Administering academic programs in higher education*. San Diego, CA: Institute for Leisure Behavior, San Diego State University.

Furnham, A. (1992). *Personality at work: The role of individual differences in the workplace*. London: Routledge.

Glassick, C., Huber, M., & Maeroff, G. (1997). *Scholarship assessed: Evaluation of the professoriate*. San Francisco: Jossey-Bass.

Keirsey, D., & Bates, M. (1998). *Please understand me, II: Temperament, character, intelligence*. Del Mar, CA: Prometheus Nemesis.

Knight, W., & Holen, M. *(1985)*. Leadership and the perceived effectiveness of department chairpersons. *Journal of Higher Education, 56*(6), 677-90.

Mawson, M. (1998). Recruitment and selection of the HPERD department chair. *The Chronicle of Physical Education in Higher Education, 9*(3), 3, 12-13, 18.

Mobley, T. (1999). The development of department chairpersons. *The Chronicle of Physical Education in Higher Education, 10*(1), 1, 10-11.

Morris, V. C. (1981). *Deaning: Middle management in academe*. Urbana, IL: University of Illinois Press.

Neff, T., & Ogden, D. (1998). Third annual route to the top: Pinball wizards. *Chief Executive*, January/February, 32-39.

References

Rosovsky, H. (1990). *The university: An owner's manual.* New York: W.W. Norton.

Seagren, A., Creswell, J., & Wheeler, D. (1993). *The department chair: New roles, responsibilities, and challenges (ASHE-ERIC Higher Education Report, no. 1).* Washington, DC: School of Education and Human Development, George Washington University.

Tucker, A. (1992). *Chairing the academic department: Leadership among peers.* New York: American Council on Education/Macmillan.

24 The Administrator's Role: Advice for the Future

Barbara A. Passmore, *Professor and Dean, Health and Human Performance, Indiana State University*

James E. Bryant, *Professor and Department Chair Emeritus, San Jose State University*

J. Laurence Passmore, *Professor, Department of Counseling, Indiana State University*

The university is no longer a sanctuary for the uninterrupted creation and dissemination of knowledge. No longer are ivy-covered walls able to protect the academy. The democratization of information, technology, and finance make it impossible for institutions of higher education to remain an island. Various stakeholders are demanding participation and accountability in ways not easily foreseen even two decades ago. Chairs and deans of health, kinesiology, and leisure-studies (HKLS) units on 21st-century campuses are greatly challenged by this notion of a university without walls.

Furthermore, the academy is one of the last institutions in the United States to "right size" and streamline its operations, and HKLS administrative personnel are now confronted with reorganization, increased faculty workloads, and a reduction in the size and quantity of their programs nationwide. As legislatures call for fiscal accountability, faculty and administrators are pressed to find and cultivate alternate funding sources. Pressure mounts to increase grant-writing efforts, create cooperative ventures with corporate and community sectors, organize fundraisers, and seek equipment donations. Distance education and "e-learning" provide new means to reach traditional and non-traditional students, yet accompanying these new opportunities are demands for technologically advanced equipment and for the professional training required to use it. HKLS administrators are confronted with a myriad of new duties, far beyond the traditional ones of overseeing budgets, handling personnel matters, meeting with student representatives, monitoring faculty performance, and scheduling meetings. The chapter authors have attempted to address the full range of administrative duties in today's complex higher-education environment and global society. We conclude with a listing of maxims representing the collected wisdom of these authors and of those who attended the 1998 College and University Administrators Council summer conference at Copper Mountain, Colorado:

"Pause" before making a decision. Sit on it. Give it serious thought.

—Charles Ash

When you face the sandstorms, thunderstorms, hailstorms, and venting storms, remain calm.

—Judith Bischoff

The most important thing you do is hire and retain excellent faculty. Spend whatever time, pain, and resources are necessary to do so.

—Judy Brookhiser

Seek council, listen, and reflect before you make a decision.

—Dana Brooks

Understand that most situations are not truly crises. So, take time to analyze and prioritize before responding.

—James Bryant

There is nothing more constant than change.

—Tony Ciccone

There is a rationale for every policy, procedure, or process. Discover the rationale, examine the validity. If valid, initiate change.

—William J. Considine

The three criteria for making a faculty appointment: "this person is honest," "this person is capable," and "this person is a team player."

—James Disch

In accepting an administrative appointment, remember your roots, the things that initially "drove" you into higher education: a passion for teaching, a sense of wonderment, and the scholarly, inquiring mind.

—John Dunn

Rule Number One: Don't ever write down that which you wouldn't say to someone face to face.
Rule Number Two: Don't ever write anything down.

—Chip East

You're never as good as you think you are, and never as bad as they say you are.

—Al Ellard

Administrative "release" time is always 25 percent short of what the job requires in "real" time.

—Keith Ernce

When in doubt, consult! When consulting, trust yourself!

—Steve Estes

"Details, details, details"—administrators need to attend to details.

—Ron Feingold

If you sit on a tack, you are better off.

—Don Franks

The buck stops here.

—Trent Gabert

Identify "high-maintenance" faculty early in their tenure/promotion period. Move them or move them out quickly.

—Sandy Gangstead

An examination of the leadership-behavior literature reveals a consistent admonition: nothing is more important than professional integrity.

—John Massengale

Personnel management is the most important aspect of a department chair's responsibilities. You are expected to fulfill promises made by your predecessor. Some will suspect you of giving advantage to faculty appointed during your term.

—Marlene Mawson

You have to have patience and good communication skills.

—Don McKillip

Never knowingly compromise your integrity.

—Alex McNeill

If you walk around, it might not come around.

—Barbara Passmore

Keep your eyes and ears on the obvious.

—J. Laurence Passmore

Become a good listener if you aren't already. Keep your conversations with faculty confidential. Be supportive and positive.

—Donna Phillips

Some days you step in it…some days you don't.

—Jan Rintala

Leadership is initially lonely. Establish collegial administrative relationships before you exhibit trust. And "to thine own self be true."

—Erika Sander

Before holding regularly scheduled faculty meetings, request agenda items and distribute them to faculty. Keep the meeting focused on the agenda. Allow 30 minutes for action items. keep meetings to one house in length.

—William Servedio

To be a successful manager: "Learn to handle hot things, keep your knives sharp, and, above all, have fun." (Julia Child)

—Steve Smidley

Always be mindful that one's reputation for integrity will usually outlive one's accomplishments or mistakes.

—Richard Swanson

"Additional problems are the offspring of poor solutions." (Mark Twain)

—Jerry Thomas

Prizes aren't awarded for predicting rain, but for building arks.

—Tom Templin

Never be surprised, never assume anything.

—Garth Tymeson

Award and reward more than necessary. Focus on performance, not the individual.

—George White

We say goodbye and good administering to you and leave you with these words found on a poster some two or more decades old: "Sometimes the better part of wisdom is to follow good advice."